Kohlhammer

Pädiatrische Neurologie

Herausgegeben von Florian Heinen

Übersicht über die bereits erschienenen Bände:
- Florian Heinen, Sandro Krieg, Ingo Borggräfe, Matthias Kieslich, Jens Böhmer, Birgit Ertl-Wagner, Alenka Pecar: Neuropharmakotherapie und klinische Systematik
  ISBN: 978-3-17-021663-1

Mirjam N. Landgraf, Florian Heinen

Fetales Alkoholsyndrom

S3-Leitlinie zur Diagnostik

Verlag W. Kohlhammer

Die Leitlinie ist eingetragen unter der AWMF-Registernummer: 022–025

Dieses Werk einschließlich aller seiner Teile ist urheberrechtlich geschützt. Jede Verwendung außerhalb der engen Grenzen des Urheberrechts ist ohne Zustimmung des Verlags unzulässig und strafbar. Das gilt insbesondere für Vervielfältigungen, Übersetzungen, Mikroverfilmungen und für die Einspeicherung und Verarbeitung in elektronischen Systemen.

Die Wiedergabe von Warenbezeichnungen, Handelsnamen und sonstigen Kennzeichen in diesem Buch berechtigt nicht zu der Annahme, dass diese von jedermann frei benutzt werden dürfen. Vielmehr kann es sich auch dann um eingetragene Warenzeichen oder sonstige geschützte Kennzeichen handeln, wenn sie nicht eigens als solche gekennzeichnet sind.

1. Auflage 2013

Alle Rechte vorbehalten
© 2013 W. Kohlhammer GmbH Stuttgart
Umschlag: Gestaltungskonzept Peter Horlacher
Umschlagabbildung: © Kathrin Schneider
Gesamtherstellung:
W. Kohlhammer Druckerei GmbH + Co. KG, Stuttgart
Printed in Germany

ISBN 978-3-17-023444-4

Inhaltsverzeichnis

Abkürzungsverzeichnis 7

Pocket Guide Fetales Alkoholsyndrom

1 Einleitung 11

2 Methodik 13
   2.1 Zusammensetzung der Leitliniengruppe 13
   2.2 Literaturrecherche und Evidenzbewertung 16
   2.3 Erstellung von Evidenztabellen 21
   2.4 Formale Konsensfindung und Formulierung von
        Empfehlungen 21
   2.5 Verabschiedung 23
   2.6 Verbreitung und Implementierung 23
   2.7 Finanzierung der Leitlinie und Darlegung möglicher
        Interessenkonflikte 25
   2.8 Gültigkeitsdauer und Aktualisierungsverfahren 25

3 Hintergrundinformationen:
   Ergebnisse der fokussierten Literaturrecherche 26
   3.1 Prävalenz von mütterlichem Alkoholkonsum in der
        Schwangerschaft und Prävalenz des Fetalen Alkohol-
        syndroms 26
   3.2 Risikofaktoren für mütterlichen Alkoholkonsum in der
        Schwangerschaft 30
   3.3 Risikofaktoren für die Entwicklung eines Fetalen Alkohol-
        syndroms 35

4 Kiterien für die Diagnose Fetales Alkoholsyndrom bei Kindern und
   Jugendlichen:
   Ergebnisse der systematischen Literaturrecherche 38
   4.1 Konsentierte Kriterien und Empfehlungen für die Diagnostik
        des FAS bei Kindern und Jugendlichen in Deutschland . . 39
   4.2 Differentialdiagnosen zum FAS bei Kindern und Jugend-
        lichen 57

Anhang 1:
Methodik Fokussierte Literaturrecherche
Hintergrundinformationen 60

Anhang 2:
Methodik Systematische Literaturrecherche
Diagnostische Kriterien 71

Anhang 3:
Evidenzklassifikationssystem nach Oxford (März 2009) 76

Anhang 4:
Evidenztabellen zur eingeschlossenen Literatur über die diagnostischen
Kriterien des FAS 79

Anhang 5:
Eingeschlossene Studien der systematischen Literaturrecherche . . . 190

Anhang 6:
Algorithmus Abklärung Fetales Alkoholsyndrom 195

Anhang 7:
Vorgeschlagene neuropsychologische Diagnostik bei Kindern und
Jugendlichen mit Verdacht auf FAS 196

Register 222

Content^PLUS
Pocket Guide Fetales Alkoholsyndrom zum Ausdrucken

Abkürzungsverzeichnis

4DDC	4-Digit Diagnostic Code
ABAS	Adaptive Behaviour System
ACOG	American Congress of Obstetricians and Gynecologists
ADD	Attention Deficit Disorder, Aufmerksamkeitsstörung, ADS
ADHD	Attention Deficit Hyperactivity Disorder, Aufmerksamkeits-Hyperaktivitätsstörung, ADHS
ADHS	Attention Deficit Hyperactivity Syndrome, Aufmerksamkeitsdefizit-Hyperaktivitäts-Syndrom
AE	Alcohol exposed, alkoholexponiert
ÄZQ	Ärztliches Zentrum für Qualität in der Medizin
ALT	Alanin-Aminotransferase
ANOVA	Analysis of Variance – Varianzanalyse
ARBD	Alcohol Related Birth Defects, alkoholbedingte Geburtsdefekte
ARND	Alcohol Related Neurodevelopmental Disorder, alkoholbedingte entwicklungsneurologische Störungen
AST	Aspartat-Aminotransferase
AUC	Area Under The Curve, unter der Kurve liegender Bereich
AWMF	Arbeitsgemeinschaft der Wissenschaftlichen Medizinischen Fachgesellschaften e. V.
BASC	Behavior Assessment System for Children
Binge Drinking	Exzessiver Alkoholkonsum zu einer Gelegenheit
BMA	British Medical Association
BMI	Body Mass Index
BRIEF	Behavior Rating Inventory of Executive Function
CANTAB	Cambridge Neuropsychological Test Automated Battery
CASL	Comprehensive Assessment of Spoken Language
CAVLT	Children´s Auditory Verbal Learning Test
CBCL	Child Behavior Checklist, Verhaltens-Fragebogen für Kinder
CD	Conduct Disorder – Verhaltensstörung
CDC	Centre of Disease Control
CDT	Carbohydrat-defizientes Transferrin
CEBM	Centre for Evidence Based Medicine
CELF	Clinical Evaluation of Language Fundamentals
CELF-P	Clinical Evaluation of Language Fundamentals – Preschool
CIFASD	Collaborative Initiative on Fetal Alcohol Spectrum Disorders
CMS	Children's Memory Scale

CNS	Central Nervous System, zentrales Nervensystem
CPM	Coloured Progressive Matrices
CRS-R	Conners' Rating Scales-Revised
CPT	Continuous Performance Test
CVLT-C	California Verbal Learning Test-Children's Version
D-KEFS	Delis Kaplan Executive Function System
DPN	Fetal Alcohol Syndrome Diagnostic And Prevention Network Diagnostic Guide
D-Score	Discriminant Score
DSM-IV	Diagnostic and Statistical Manual of Mental Disorders – Diagnostisches und Statistisches Manual mentaler Störungen
DSS-ROCF	Diagnostic Scoring System-Rey-Osterrieth Complex Figure
DTI	Diffusion Tensor Imaging
EEG	Elektroencephalographie
ELT	Expressive Language Test
EMBASE	Excerpta Medica Database
EP	Evozierte Potentiale
EVT	Expressive Vocabulary Test
FABS	Fetal Alcohol Behavior Scale
FAEE	Fatty acids ethyl ester, Fettsäure-Äthyl-Ester
FAS	Fetal Alcohol Syndrome – Fetales Alkoholsyndrom
FASD	Fetal Alcohol Spectrum Disorders, Fetale Alkohol-Spektrum-Störungen
FASDC	Fetal Alcohol Syndrome Diagnostic Checklist
FSIQ	Full Scale Intelligence Quotient
FU	Follow Up
GAC	General Adaptive Composite
GC-FID	Gas Chromatography/Flame Ionization Detection
GC-MS	Gas Chromatography/Mass Spectroscopy
GGT	Gamma Glutamyl Transferase
HTA	Health Technology Assessment
IED	Intra-Extra-Dimensional Set Shift
IOM	Institute of Medicine, USA
IPDA	Questionario Osservativo per L'Identificazione Precoce delle Difficoltà di Apprendimento, italienischer standardisierter Fragebogen zur Identifikation von Lernschwierigkeiten
IQ	Intelligenzquotient
IVA CPT	Integrated Visual and Auditory Continuous Performance Test
LoE	Level of Evidence – Evidenzlevel
LMU	Ludwig-Maximilians-Universität München
LPA	Latent Profile Analysis

MCV	Mittleres korpuskuläres Volumen
MD	Mean Diameter, mittlerer Durchmesser
Movement ABC	Movement Assessment Battery for Children
MRI	Magnetic Resonance Imaging
MRS	Magnetresonanzspektroskopie
MRT	Magnetresonanztomographie
ND	Neurobehavioural Disorder, Verhaltensstörung
NEPSY	Developmental NEuroPSYchological Assessment, Battery of Tests
NHMRC	National Health and Medical Research Council
NHS	National Health Service
ODD	Oppositional Defiant Disorder, oppositionell aufsässige Verhaltensstörung
OFC	Occipital Frontal Circumference, (fronto-occipitaler) Kopfumfang
OWLS	Oral and Written Language Scales
PA	Pairs Associate
PAE	Prenatal Alcohol Exposure, pränatale Alkoholexposition
PAUI	Prenatal Alcohol Use Interview
PEA	Prenatal Exposure to Alcohol, pränatale Alkoholexposition
PF	Palpebral Fissure, Lidspalte
PFAS	partial FAS – Partielles Fetales Alkoholsyndrom
PFL	Palpebral Fissure Length, Lidspalten-Länge
PLAI	Preschool Language Assessment Instrument
PPVT	Peabody Picture Vocabulary Test
PPW	Positiver Prädiktiver Wert
RCFT	Rey Complex Figure Test
REM	Rapid Eye Movement, schnelle Augenbewegungen
ROC	Receiver Operator Characteristics
SD	Standard Deviation, Standardabweichung
SE	Static Encephalopathy, statische Encephalopathie
SES	Socioeconomic Status, sozio-ökonomischer Status
SIM	Selected Ion Monitoring
SSP	Short sensory Profile
T-ACE	Alkohol-Screening-Test (4 Fragen)
TLC	Test of Language Competence
TNL	Test of Narrative Language
TOLD-I	Test of Language Development-Intermediate
TOLD-P	Test of Language Development-Primary
TONI	Test of Nonverbal Intelligence
TOPS	Test of Problem Solving
TOWK	Test of Word Knowledge
TWEAK	Alkohol-Screening-Test (5 Fragen)

VDRL	Visual Discrimination Reversal Learning Test
VMI	Visual-Motor Integration, visuell-motorische Integration
VRAT	Wide Range Achievement Test
WBAA	Whole Blood-Associated Acetaldehyde
WCST	Wisconsin Card Sorting Test
WIAT	Wechsler Individual Achievement Test
WISC	Wechsler Intelligence Scale for Children
WISC-R	Wechsler Intelligence Scale for Children Revised
WPPSI-R	Wechsler Preschool and Primary Scale of Intelligence
WRAT	Wide Range Achievement Test
ZNS	Zentrales Nervensystem

POCKET GUIDE FAS MIRJAM N. LANDGRAF & FLORIAN HEINEN

THINK KIDS

**DON´T DRINK
STOP FAS** Fetales Alkohol Syndrom

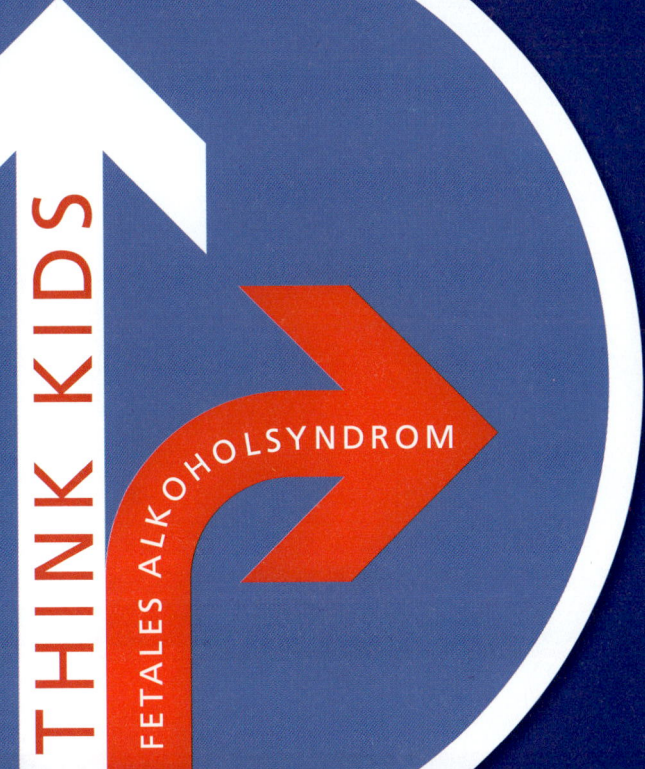

MÖGLICHE RISIKOFAKTOREN FÜR DIE ENTWICKLUNG EINES FAS

ALKOHOL- UND DROGENKONSUM DER MUTTER
- Hoher Alkoholkonsum
- Chronischer Alkoholkonsum
- Alkoholkonsum im 1. und 2. Trimenon im Gegensatz zu Alkoholkonsum ausschließlich im 3. Trimenon
- Alkoholkonsum während der gesamten Schwangerschaft
- Zusätzliche Einnahme von Amphetaminen oder multiplen Drogen

MÜTTERLICHE RISIKOFAKTOREN
- Alter > 30 Jahre
- Spezifische ethnische Zugehörigkeit
- Geringer sozioökonomischer Status
- Mütterliche Unterernährung, Mangel an Spurenelementen oder Vitaminen
- Stress
- Geburtshilfliche Komplikationen
- Geschwister mit FASD
- Genetischer Hintergrund

4 DIAGNOSTISCHE SÄULEN DES FAS

Zur Diagnose eines FAS **sollten alle** Kriterien 1 bis 4 zutreffen:

1 WACHSTUMSAUFFÄLLIGKEITEN

2 FACIALE AUFFÄLLIGKEITEN

3 ZNS AUFFÄLLIGKEITEN

4 BESTÄTIGTE ODER NICHT BESTÄTIGTE INTRAUTERINE ALKOHOL-EXPOSITION

Bei Kontakt zum Gesundheits- und Hilfesystem sollten, wenn ein Kind Auffälligkeiten in einer der vier diagnostischen Säulen zeigt, die drei anderen diagnostischen Säulen beurteilt oder ihre Beurteilung veranlasst werden.

DIFFERENTIALDIAGNOSEN

1. WACHSTUMSSTÖRUNGEN

1.1. PRÄNATALE WACHSTUMSSTÖRUNGEN

1.1.1. UNGESTÖRTE INTRAUTERINE VERSORGUNG
FETALE PATHOLOGIE
ENDOGEN
- Fehlbildungen
- Genetische Syndrome (z.B. Turner-Syndrom, Silver-Russell-Syndrom)
- Stoffwechselerkrankungen

EXOGEN
- Intrauterine Infektionen z.B. Röteln, Cytomegalie, Toxoplasmose, Herpes simplex, HIV, EBV, Parvo B19
- Strahlenexposition

1.1.2. GESTÖRTE INTRAUTERINE VERSORGUNG
PRÄPLAZENTAR
MATERNALE ERKRANKUNGEN
- Präeklampsie, Hypotonie, Anämie, zyanotische Vitien, Kollagenosen, chronische Nierenerkrankungen
- Toxische Einflüsse, Nikotin, Drogen
- Erhöhte maternale psychosoziale Belastung

PLAZENTAR
- Plazenta praevia
- Gestörte Plazentation (Uterusfehlbildung, Myome)
- Auf die Plazenta beschränkte Chromosomenstörung

1.2. POSTNATALE WACHSTUMSSTÖRUNGEN
- Familiärer Kleinwuchs
- Konstitutionelle Entwicklungsverzögerung
- Skelettdysplasien (z.B. Hypochondroplasie, Achondroplasie, Osteogenesis imperfecta)
- Metabolische Störungen
- Renale Erkrankungen
- Hormonelle Störungen
- Genetische Syndrome (z.B. Trisomie 21)
- Chronische Erkrankungen
- Malabsorption oder Mangelernährung (v.a. Mangel an Vit. D, Calcium, Eiweiß, generelle Unterernährung)
- Psychosozialer Kleinwuchs

Zur Erfüllung des Kriteriums
WACHSTUMSAUFFÄLLIGKEITEN

soll mindestens 1 der folgenden Auffälligkeiten, adaptiert an Gestationsalter, Alter, Geschlecht, dokumentiert zu einem beliebigen Zeitpunkt, zutreffen:

(1) **Geburts- oder Körpergewicht** ≤ 10. Perzentile
(2) **Geburts- oder Körperlänge** ≤ 10. Perzentile
(3) **Body Mass Index** ≤ 10. Perzentile

Zu Mikrocephalie siehe 3.2

DIFFERENTIALDIAGNOSEN

2. FACIALE AUFFÄLLIGKEITEN
2.1. TOXISCHE EFFEKTE IN DER SCHWANGERSCHAFT
- Antikonvulsiva
- Toluol
- Maternale Phenylketonurie

2.2. GENETISCH BEDINGTE ERKRANKUNGEN
- Aarskog-Syndrom
- Cornelia-de-Lange-Syndrom
- Dubowitz-Syndrom
- Noonan-Syndrom
- Williams-Beuren-Syndrom (Mikrodeletion 7q11.23)
- Di-George-Syndrom (VCFS) (Mikrodeletion 22q11)
- Blepharophimosis-Syndrom
- Hallermann-Streiff-Syndrom
- 3-M-Syndrom
- Smith-Lemli-Opitz-Syndrom
- SHORT-Syndrom
- Feingold-Syndrom (Trisomie 9)
- Kabuki-Syndrom
- Peters-Plus-Syndrom
- Rubinstein-Taybi-Syndrom
- Geleophysic Dysplasia

Zur Erfüllung des Kriteriums
FACIALE AUFFÄLLIGKEITEN

sollen alle 3 facialen Anomalien vorhanden sein:

(1) **Kurze Lidspalten** (≤ 3. Perzentile)

(2) **Verstrichenes Philtrum**
 (Rang IV oder V Lip-Philtrum-Guide)

(3) **Schmale Oberlippe**
 (Rang IV oder V Lip-Philtrum-Guide)

Lip-Philtrum-Guide

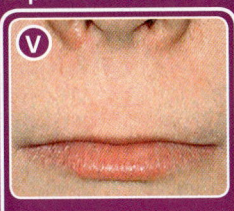
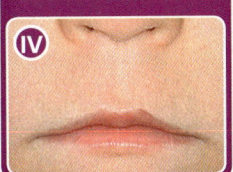
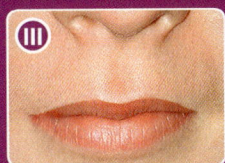
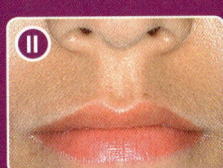
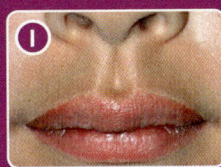

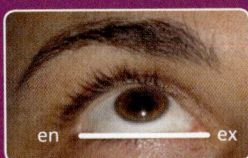
Messung der Lidspaltenlänge

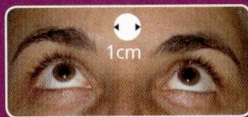
Referenzpunkt Lidspaltenlänge

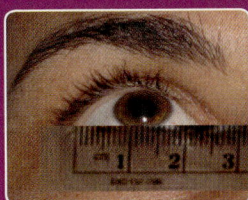
Lineal-Messung Lidspaltenlänge

© Mirjam N. Landgraf,
University of Munich, Germany

© Susan Astley,
University of Washington, USA

DIFFERENTIALDIAGNOSEN

3. ZNS-AUFFÄLLIGKEITEN
3.1. FUNKTIONELLE ZNS-AUFFÄLLIGKEITEN
- Kombinierte umschriebene Entwicklungsstörung
- Intelligenzminderung unterschiedlichen Grades
- Umschriebene Entwicklungsstörung des Sprechens und der Sprache
- Umschriebene Entwicklungsstörung motorischer Funktionen
- Umschriebene Entwicklungsstörung schulischer Fertigkeiten
- Einfache Aufmerksamkeits- und Aktivitätsstörung
- Hyperkinetische Störung des Sozialverhaltens
- Störung des Sozialverhaltens mit oppositionellem, aufsässigem Verhalten
- Kombinierte Störung des Sozialverhaltens und der Emotionen
- Stereotypien
- Aggressivität
- Delinquenz
- Suchterkrankungen
- Reaktive Bindungsstörung des Kindesalters
- Posttraumatische Belastungsstörung
- Sexuelle Verhaltensabweichung
- Schlafstörungen
- Angststörung/Panikstörung
- Affektive Störung/Depressive Störung
- Epilepsien anderer Genese

3.2. MIKROCEPHALIE
- Familiäre Mikrocephalie
- Genetische Syndrome (siehe 2.2)
- Pränatale Mangelversorgung, toxische Schädigung, Infektion
- Hypoxisch-ischämische Hirnschädigung
- Maternale Erkrankungen
- Postnatale Mangelernährung
- Stoffwechselstörungen
- Chronische Erkrankungen

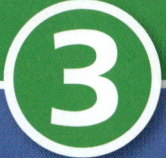

Zur Erfüllung des Kriteriums
ZNS–AUFFÄLLIGKEITEN

sollte 3.1 oder/und **3.2** zutreffen:

 Zur Erfüllung des Kriteriums
FUNKTIONELLE ZNS-AUFFÄLLIGKEITEN

sollte mindestens 1 der folgenden Auffälligkeiten zutreffen, die nicht adäquat für das Alter ist und nicht allein durch den familiären Hintergrund oder das soziale Umfeld erklärt werden kann:

(1) Globale Intelligenzminderung mindestens 2 Standardabweichungen unterhalb der Norm
oder signifikante kombinierte Entwicklungs-verzögerung bei Kindern unter 2 Jahren

(2) Leistung mindestens 2 Standardabweichungen unterhalb der Norm
entweder in mindestens 3 der folgenden Bereiche
oder in mindestens 2 der folgenden Bereiche in Kombination mit Epilepsie:
Sprache
Feinmotorik
Räumlich-visuelle Wahrnehmung oder räumlich-konstruktive Fähigkeiten
Lern- oder Merkfähigkeit
Exekutive Funktionen
Rechenfertigkeiten
Aufmerksamkeit
Soziale Fertigkeiten oder Verhalten

 Zur Erfüllung des Kriteriums
STRUKTURELLE ZNS-AUFFÄLLIGKEITEN

sollte folgende Auffälligkeit, adaptiert an Gestationsalter, Alter, Geschlecht, dokumentiert zu einem beliebigen Zeitpunkt, zutreffen:

Mikrocephalie
(≤ 10. Perzentile/≤ 3. Perzentile, siehe Leitlinie)

MÖGLICHE RISIKOFAKTOREN FÜR MÜTTERLICHEN ALKOHOLKONSUM WÄHREND DER SCHWANGERSCHAFT

ALTER
- > 30 Jahre
- binge drinking < 27 Jahre

NATIONALITÄT
- kein Migrationshintergrund
- hohe Akkulturation
- spezifische Minderheiten (z.B. Native Indians, Inuit)

GESUNDHEITSBEZOGENE RISIKOFAKTOREN
- Beginn von Alkoholkonsum in einem frühen Lebensalter
- Alkoholkonsum und insbesondere binge drinking vor der Schwangerschaft
- vorherige Therapie wegen Alkoholproblemen
- Konsum illegaler Drogen
- Rauchen

SCHWANGERSCHAFTSBESONDERHEITEN
- ungeplante oder ungewollte Schwangerschaft
- wenig oder späte pränatale Vorsorge

SOZIOÖKONOMISCHER STATUS
- Hoher sozioökonomischer Status
- Erhalten öffentlicher Zuwendungen (USA)

SOZIALE UMGEBUNG
- Single oder unverheiratet
- Alkohol- oder Drogenkonsum in der Familie oder beim Partner
- Geringe soziale Unterstützung

PSYCHISCHE FAKTOREN
- Stattgefundene oder aktuelle körperliche Misshandlung oder sexueller Missbrauch durch Partner oder Fremden
- Psychische und psychiatrische Störungen inkl. Depression, Angststörung, Panikstörung, sexuelle Funktionsstörungen

④ BESTÄTIGTE ODER NICHT BESTÄTIGTE INTRAUTERINE ALKOHOL-EXPOSITION

Wenn Auffälligkeiten in den drei übrigen diagnostischen Säulen bestehen, **soll** die Diagnose eines Fetalen Alkoholsyndroms auch **ohne** Bestätigung eines mütterlichen Alkoholkonsums während der Schwangerschaft gestellt werden.

MÖGLICHE ANLAUFSTELLEN FÜR MENSCHEN MIT FASD

ambulant
- FASD-Zentrum Charité Berlin
  Hr. Prof. Dr. med. Hans-Ludwig Spohr
  Fr. Dipl.-Psych. Jessica Wagner   fasd-zentrum@charite.de
- Evangelischer Verein Sonnenhof
  Fr. Dipl.-Psych. Gela Becker   sonnenhof-ev@t-online.de
- Universität Münster
  Hr. Dr. phil. Dipl.-Psych. Reinhold Feldmann   feldrei@uni-muenster.de
- Klinikum der Universität München
  Dr. von Haunersches Kinderspital
  iSPZ München TESS-Ambulanz www.spz-muenchen.info
  Fr. Dr. med. Dipl.-Psych. Mirjam N. Landgraf
  mirjam.landgraf@med.uni-muenchen.de
- Heckscher Klinikum München (Kinder- und Jugendpsychiatrie, Psychosomatik und Psychotherapie)
  Hr. Dr. med. Martin Sobanski   martin.sobanski@heckscher-klinik.de
  Fr. Dipl.-Psych. Penelope Thomas
  penelope.thomas@heckscher-klinik.de
- Elisabeth Krankenhaus Essen, SPZ
  Dr. med. Antje Erencin   spz@contilia.de
- LVR Klinikum Essen (Kinder- und Jugendpsychiatrie, Psychotherapie und Psychosomatik),
  Universität Duisburg-Essen
  http://www.rk-essen.lvr.de/behandlungsangebote/ambulanzen/fas.htm
  Dr. med. Nora Dörrie   Nora.Doerrie@lvr.de
  Dipl.-Psych. Inga Freunscht   Inga.Freunscht@lvr.de
- Sozialpädiatrische Zentren
- Kinder- und Jugendärzte

stationär
- KMG Rehabilitationszentrum Sülzhayn
  Fr. Dr. med. Heike Hoff-Emden   h.hoff-emden@kmg-kliniken.de

juristisch
- Fr. Gila Schindler
  Rechtsanwältin für Kinder- und Jugendhilferecht   schindler@msbh.de

INFORMATION

Diagnostik des Fetalen Alkoholsyndroms
Kurzfassung, Langfassung und Leitlinienbericht
www.awmf.org

Rückfragen
Gesellschaft für Neuropädiatrie (GNP)
info@neuropaediatrie.com

Internationale Leitlinien zu FASD

1. Astley, S. 2004. Diagnostic Guide for Fetal Alcohol Spectrum Disorders: The 4-Digit Diagnostic Code. University of Washington Publication Services
2. National Centre on Birth Defects and Developmental Disabilities. Fetal Alcohol Syndrome: Guidelines for Referral and Diagnosis. 2004. Centre for Disease Control
3. Hoyme HE et al. A practical clinical approach to diagnosis of fetal alcohol spectrum disorders: Clarification of the 1996 Institute of Medicine Criteria. Paediatrics 2005; 115: 47
4. Chudley A et al. Fetal alcohol spectrum disorder: Canadian guidelines for diagnosis. Can Med Assoc J 2005; 172 (Suppl) sowie deren Aktualisierung 2008 (Goh et al., 2008)

Selbsthilfegruppe FASD Deutschland e.V.
www.fasd-deutschland.de

Homepage der Drogenbeauftragten
www.drogenbeauftragte.de

Bundeszentrale für gesundheitliche Aufklärung
www.bzga.de

Expertinnen / Experten	Funktion
Dipl.-Psych. Gela Becker	Fachliche Leiterin Evangelisches Kinderheim Sonnenhof
Dr. med. Beate Erbas	Bayerische Akademie für Sucht- und Gesundheitsfragen
Dr. Dipl.-Psych. Reinhold Feldmann	FASD-Zentrum Universität Münster
PD Dr. med. Anne Hilgendorff	Neonatologie und Neuropädiatrie, Universität München (LMU)
Dr. med. Heike Hoff-Emden	Chefärztin KMG Rehabilitationszentrum Sülzhayn
Dr. med. Ulrike Horacek	Vorstandsmitglied der DGSPJ, Gesundheitsamt Recklinghausen
Prof. Dr. med. Ina Kopp	Leiterin AWMF-IMWi
Dr. med. Dipl.-Psych. Mirjam N. Landgraf	Neuropädiatrie, FASD-Ambulanz, iSPZ, Universität München (LMU)
Gisela Michalowski	Vorsitzende der Patientenvertretung FASD Deutschland e.V.
Veerle Moubax	Vorstand der Patientenvertretung FASD Deutschland e.V.
Dr. Monika Nothacker	ÄZQ
Carla Pertl	Stadtjugendamt München
Dr. Eva Rehfueß	IBE, Universität München (LMU)
Dr. med. Monika Reincke	Referat für Gesundheit und Umwelt der Landeshauptstadt München, Gesundheitsvorsorge für Kinder und Jugendliche
Andreas Rösslein	Neonatologie, Universität München (LMU)
Gila Schindler	Rechtsanwältin für Kinder- und Jugendhilferecht
Prof. Dr. med. Andreas Schulze	Leiter der Neonatologie, Universität München (LMU)
Dr. med. Martin Sobanski	Kinder- und Jugendpsychiatrie, FASD-Ambulanz, Heckscher Klinikum, München
Prof. Dr. med. Hans-Ludwig Spohr	FASD-Zentrum, Charité Berlin
Dipl.-Psych. Penelope Thomas	Kinder- und Jugendpsychiatrie, FASD-Ambulanz, Heckscher Klinikum, München
Dipl.-Psych. Jessica Wagner	FASD-Zentrum, Charité Berlin
Dr. med. Wendelina Wendenburg	Vorstand der Patientenvertretung FASD Deutschland e.V.

Realisation
Bundesministerium für Gesundheit www.bmg.bund.de
Drogenbeauftragte der Bundesregierung
Fr. Dr. M. Dyckmans www.drogenbeauftragte.de
Deutsche Gesellschaft für Kinder- und Jugendmedizin www.dgkj.de
Gesellschaft für Neuropädiatrie www.neuropaediatrie.com
Klinikum der Universität München Dr. von Haunersches Kinderspital
Pädiatrische Neurologie, Entwicklungsneurologie und Sozialpädiatrie
iSPZ München www.spz-muenchen.com

Design Kathrin Schneider, München www.grafikschneider.de
Copyright Mirjam N. Landgraf & Florian Heinen, München

Gefördert durch:
Bundesministerium für Gesundheit

aufgrund eines Beschlusses des Deutschen Bundestages

IMPRESSUM

Autoren der Leitlinie
Dr. med. Dipl.-Psych. Mirjam N. Landgraf
Prof. Dr. med. Florian Heinen

Organisation der Leitlinienentwicklung
Dr. med. Dipl.-Psych. Mirjam N. Landgraf (Leitlinienkoordination,
  Literaturrecherche, Moderation und Leitlinien-Sekretariat)
  Dr. von Haunersches Kinderspital, LMU München
Prof. Dr. med. Florian Heinen (Leitlinienkoordination und Moderation)
  Dr. von Haunersches Kinderspital, LMU München
  DGKJ & GNP
Dr. med. Monika Nothacker (Literaturrecherche und Evidenzbewertung)
  Ärztliches Zentrum für Qualität in der Medizin (ÄZQ)
Prof. Dr. med. Ina Kopp (Methodische Führung und Moderation)
  Arbeitsgemeinschaft der Wissenschaftlichen Medizinischen Fachgesellschaften e.V. (AWMF)
Dr. Sandra Dybowski (Organisatorische Unterstützung und Ansprechpartnerin im BMG)
Dr. Tilmann Holzer (Ansprechpartner in der Geschäftsstelle der Drogenbeauftragten)

Beteiligte Fachgesellschaften / Berufsverbände /	MandatsträgerInnen
Deutsche Gesellschaft für Kinder- und Jugendmedizin	Prof. Dr. med. Florian Heinen
Gesellschaft für Neuropädiatrie	Prof. Dr. med. Florian Heinen
Deutsche Gesellschaft für Sozialpädiatrie und Jugendmedizin	Prof. Dr. med. Michael Straßburg Dr. med. Juliane Spiegler
Deutsche Gesellschaft für Gynäkologie und Geburtshilfe	Prof. Dr. med. Franz Kainer
Gesellschaft für Neonatologie und Pädiatrische Intensivmedizin	Prof. Dr. med. Rolf F. Maier
Deutsche Gesellschaft für Kinder- und Jugendpsychiatrie, Psychosomatik und Psychotherapie	Prof. Dr. med. Frank Häßler
Deutsche Gesellschaft für Suchtforschung und Suchttherapie	Dr. med. Regina Rasenack
Deutsche Gesellschaft für Suchtpsychologie	Prof. Dr. Dipl.-Psych. Tanja Hoff
Deutsche Gesellschaft für Suchtmedizin	PD Dr. med. Gerhard Reymann
Deutsche Gesellschaft für Hebammenwissenschaft	Prof. Dr. rer. medic. Rainhild Schäfers
Deutscher Hebammenverband	Regine Gresens
Berufsverband der deutschen Psychologinnen und Psychologen	Dipl.-Psych. Laszlo A. Pota
Berufsverband der Kinder- und Jugendärzte	Dr. Dr. med. Nikolaus Weissenrieder
Bundesverband der Ärztinnen und Ärzte des Öffentlichen Gesundheitsdienstes	Dr. med. Gabriele Trost-Brinkhues

ALGORITHMUS
ABKLÄRUNG FETALES ALKOHOLSYNDROM

Gesundheits- und Hilfesystem

Mögliche Diagnose Fetales Alkoholsyndrom

↓

Überweisung zu FAS-erfahrenem Leistungserbringer

Mindestens 1 Wachstums-Auffälligkeit:
1. Geburts- oder Körpergewicht ≤ 10. Perzentile **oder**
2. Geburts- oder Körperlänge ≤ 10. Perzentile **oder**
3. Body Mass Index ≤ 10. Perzentile

adaptiert an Gestationsalter, Alter, Geschlecht, dokumentiert zu einem beliebigen Zeitpunkt

UND

Alle 3 für FAS typischen facialen Auffälligkeiten:
1. Kurze Lidspalten ≤ 3. Perzentile **und**
2. Verstrichenes Philtrum (Rang IV oder V Lip-Philtrum-Guide) **und**
3. Schmale Oberlippe (Rang IV oder V Lip-Philtrum-Guide)

UND

Mindestens 1 ZNS-Auffälligkeit:
1. Mikrocephalie adaptiert an Gestationsalter, Alter, Geschlecht, dokumentiert zu einem beliebigen Zeitpunkt **oder**
2. Globale Intelligenzminderung ≤ 2 Standardabweichungen oder globale Entwicklungsverzögerung bei Kindern ≤ 2 Jahre **oder**
3. Leistung ≤ 2 Standardabweichungen entweder in mindestens 3 Bereichen oder in mindestens 2 Bereichen in Kombination mit Epilepsie:
- Sprache
- Feinmotorik
- Räumlich-visuelle Wahrnehmung oder räumlich-konstruktive Fähigkeiten
- Exekutive Funktionen
- Rechenfertigkeiten
- Lern- oder Merkfähigkeit
- Aufmerksamkeit
- Soziale Fertigkeiten oder Verhalten

DIAGNOSE FAS?

JA → entsprechende Förderung

NEIN → Beobachtung und Dokumentation von Körpermaßen, Entwicklung, Kognition, Verhalten und FAS typischen Sekundärerkrankungen

1 Einleitung

Mütterlicher Alkoholkonsum während der Schwangerschaft führt häufig zu Schäden beim ungeborenen Kind. Intrauterine Alkoholexposition kann Auffälligkeiten des Wachstums, cranio-faciale, cardiale, renale, ossäre und okuläre Malformationen, Störungen der Entwicklung, der Kognition und des Verhaltens sowie Einschränkungen in Teilleistungen und somit globale Einschränkungen im Alltag bewirken. Schädigungen, die durch intrauterine Alkoholexposition hervorgerufen werden, werden unter dem Oberbegriff Fetale Alkoholspektrumstörungen (FASD, fetal alcohol spectrum disorders) zusammengefasst. Zu den Fetalen Alkoholspektrumstörungen gehören das Vollbild der Fetalen Alkoholspektrumstörungen, das sogenannte Fetale Alkoholsyndrom (FAS, fetal alcohol syndrome), das Partielle Fetale Alkoholsyndrom (pFAS, partial fetal alcohol syndrome), die Alkoholbedingte Entwicklungsneurologische Störung (ARND, alcohol related neurodevelopmental disorder) und die Alkoholbedingten Geburtsdefekte (ARBD, alcohol related birth defects).

Die vorliegende S3-Leitlinie zur Diagnostik des Fetalen Alkoholsyndroms gibt erstmalig im deutschsprachigen Raum evidenz- und konsensbasierte Empfehlungen bezüglich diagnostischer Kriterien für das *Vollbild des Fetalen Alkoholsyndroms (FAS)* bei Kindern und Jugendlichen (0 bis 18 Jahre) ab.

Aus Machbarkeitsgründen beschränkt sich die vorliegende Leitlinie auf das Vollbild FAS einerseits und die Diagnose andererseits. Sie versteht sich als ein erster Schritt auf dem notwendigen Weg zu einer umfassenden Bearbeitung auch der (noch) nicht bearbeiteten Felder der Fetalen Alkoholspektrumstörungen und der Therapie im Rahmen weiterer Leitlinien. Die deutlichen negativen Folgen intrauteriner Alkoholexposition im Erwachsenenleben, z. B. auf die Selbständigkeit und Arbeitsfähigkeit, sind hierbei ein weiteres wichtiges Thema.

Das Fetale Alkoholsyndrom entspricht einem sogenannten hirnorganischen Psychosyndrom oder einer sogenannten statischen Encephalopathie. Dabei ist jedoch zu beachten, dass die cerebrale Schädigung durch intrauterine Alkoholexposition zwar statisch ist, die Funktions- und Alltagsbeeinträchtigung der betroffenen Kinder jedoch durch frühe und individuelle Förderung deutlich beeinflussbar sind und das FAS damit die klassischen Kriterien einer „developmental disorder" aufweist.

Durch die festgelegten diagnostischen Kriterien eines FAS soll das Störungsbild früh erfasst und eine entsprechende Therapie und Förderung des Kindes initiiert werden. Dadurch kann das Auftreten sekundärer Erkrankungen von Kindern mit FAS vermindert werden.

Die Gesundheitsdienste und die Bevölkerung in Deutschland sollen über die schwerwiegenden Folgen des Alkoholkonsums während der Schwangerschaft aufgeklärt werden. Langfristig soll die Prävalenz von Alkoholkonsum in der Schwangerschaft und die Inzidenz von FAS in Deutschland reduziert werden.

Alle bisherigen Leitlinien (eine kanadische und drei amerikanische Leitlinien) beinhalten die vier diagnostischen Säulen: (1) Wachstumsauffälligkeiten, (2) faciale Auffälligkeiten, (3) ZNS-Auffälligkeiten und (4) Alkoholkonsum der Mutter während der Schwangerschaft. Von diesen internationalen Leitlinien für die Diagnose des FAS erfüllt keine die methodischen Voraussetzungen einer S3-Leitlinie. Das am besten standardisierte Diagnostikinstrument, der 4-Digit Diagnostic Code, gewichtet die vier Diagnostik-Säulen jeweils auf einer 4-Punkt-Likert-Skala und beinhaltet einen Lip-Philtrum Guide, anhand dessen man zwei der drei für FAS typischen facialen Merkmale gewichten kann. Der 4-Digit Diagnostic Code basiert nicht auf einer objektiven Literaturrecherche mit formaler Evidenzbewertung und ist aufgrund seiner Komplexität in der deutschen Praxis nicht ausreichend etabliert.

In Deutschland besteht die Notwendigkeit, standardisierte und transdisziplinäre diagnostische Kriterien für das Fetale Alkoholsyndrom zu definieren, die in der Praxis effektiv und unmissverständlich genutzt werden können.

Das Bundesministerium für Gesundheit hat daher ein Projekt (STOP-FAS) zur Erstellung einer diagnostischen Leitlinie des Fetalen Alkoholsyndroms für Deutschland initiiert, das von der Deutschen Gesellschaft für Kinder- und Jugendmedizin angenommen und dessen Federführung der Gesellschaft für Neuropädiatrie übertragen wurde.

Dieses Projekt wurde von Dr. med. Dipl.-Psych. Mirjam N. Landgraf und Prof. Dr. med. Florian Heinen im Dr. von Haunerschen Kinderspital der Ludwig-Maximilians-Universität München, in der Abteilung für Pädiatrische Neurologie, Entwicklungsneurologie und Sozialpädiatrie (integriertes Sozialpädiatrisches Zentrum, iSPZ München) geleitet.

Die Anwenderzielgruppe der Leitlinie beinhaltet personell und strukturell:

- niedergelassene sowie ambulant oder in der Klinik tätige Ärztinnen und Ärzte der folgenden Gebiete und Schwerpunkte: Gynäkologie und Geburtshilfe, Kinder- und Jugendmedizin, Neonatologie, Neuropädiatrie, Entwicklungsneurologie und Sozialpädiatrie, Kinder- und Jugendpsychiatrie, Psychotherapie und Psychosomatik, Allgemeinmedizin, Suchtmedizin und öffentlicher Gesundheitsdienst einschließlich des Schulärztlichen Dienstes.
- Niedergelassene und in der Klinik tätige Kinder- und Jugendlichen-Psychotherapeuten sowie Diplom- und Master-Psychologen
- Hebammen
- Physio-, Ergo- und Sprachtherapeuten
- Sozialpädagogen, Sozialarbeiter, Sozialhelfer
- Sozialpädiatrische Zentren
- FAS-Spezialambulanzen und FAS-Spezialisten

2 Methodik

2.1 Zusammensetzung der Leitliniengruppe

Die Organisation der Leitlinienentwicklung übernahmen:

- Dr. med. Dipl.-Psych. Mirjam N. Landgraf: Leitlinienkoordination, Literaturrecherche, Moderation und Leitlinien-Sekretariat
- Prof. Dr. med. Florian Heinen: Leitlinienkoordination und Moderation
- Dr. med. Monika Nothacker MPH: Literaturrecherche und Evidenzbewertung
- Prof. Dr. med. Ina Kopp: Methodische Führung und Moderation
- Dr. Sandra Dybowski: Organisatorische Unterstützung und Ansprechpartnerin im BMG
- Dr. Tilmann Holzer: Ansprechpartner in der Geschäftsstelle der Drogenbeauftragten

Eine Münchner Steuergruppe wurde gebildet, deren Aufgaben die fokussierte Literaturrecherche hinsichtlich der Hintergrundinformationen der Leitlinie, die Formulierung von Schlüsselfragen und Empfehlungen sowie die Diskussion möglicher Hindernisse bei der Umsetzung der Leitlinieninhalte umfasste.

Die Leitliniengruppe wurde von den Koordinatoren einberufen. Gemäß den AWMF-Vorgaben wurde sie multidisziplinär und für den Adressatenkreis repräsentativ zusammengesetzt. Die Vorstände der Fachgesellschaften und Berufsverbände nominierten Experten zur inhaltlichen Arbeit an der Leitlinie und bestätigten deren Stimmrecht für die Konsentierung der Leitlinieninhalte (Mandat). Das Projekt wurde im Juni 2011 über das Anmelderegister der AWMF im Internet öffentlich ausgeschrieben, um interessierten Gruppen eine Beteiligung zu ermöglichen.

Die Leitliniengruppe beinhaltete zusätzlich zu den Mandatsträgern der sich mit dem Krankheitsbild FAS auseinandersetzenden deutschen Fachgesellschaften und Berufsverbänden auch Experten und Patientenvertreter (▶ Abb 2.1 und ▶ Tab. 2.1 und 2.2).

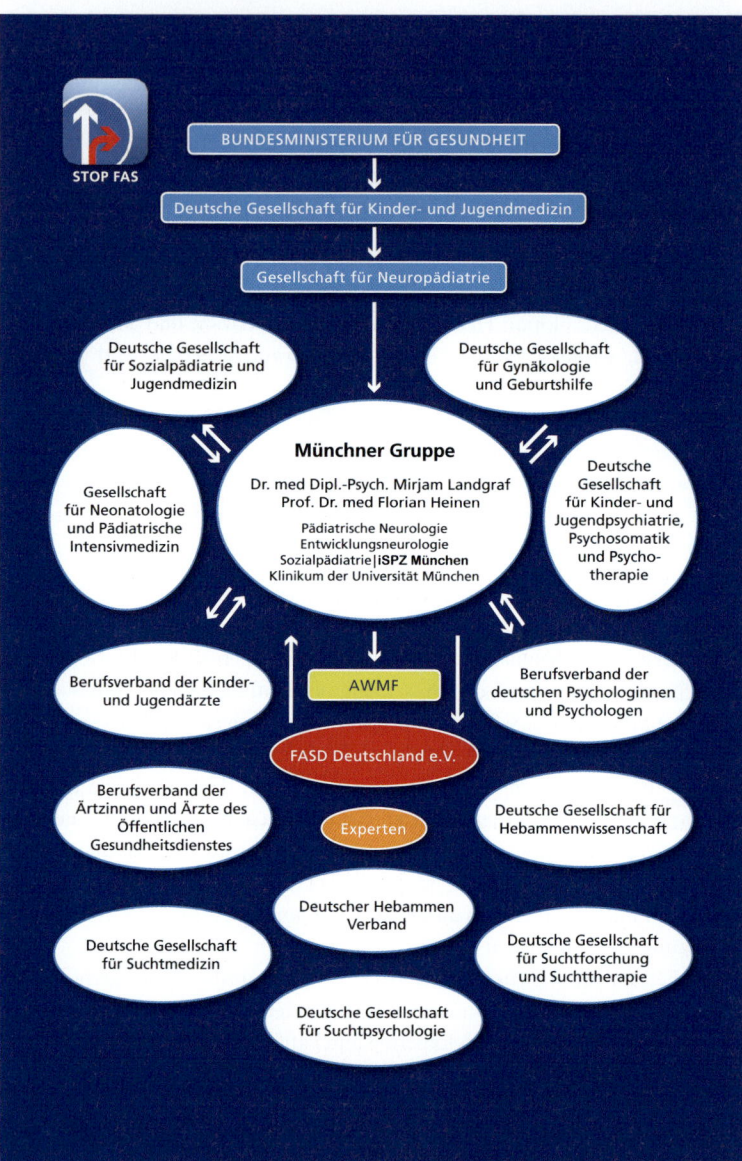

Abb. 2.1: Schaubild über die Teilnehmer am Leitlinienprojekt

Tab. 2.1: Am Leitlinienprojekt beteiligte Fachgesellschaften und Berufsverbände

Beteiligte Fachgesellschaften/Berufsverbände	Mandatsträger- und trägerinnen
Deutsche Gesellschaft für Kinder- und Jugendmedizin	Prof. Dr. med. Florian Heinen
Gesellschaft für Neuropädiatrie	Prof. Dr. med. Florian Heinen
Deutsche Gesellschaft für Sozialpädiatrie und -Jugendmedizin	Dr. med. Juliane Spiegler
Deutsche Gesellschaft für Gynäkologie und Geburtshilfe	Prof. Dr. med. Franz Kainer
Gesellschaft für Neonatologie und Pädiatrische Intensivmedizin	Prof. Dr. med. Rolf F. Maier
Deutsche Gesellschaft für Kinder- und Jugendpsychiatrie, Psychosomatik und Psychotherapie	Prof. Dr. med. Frank Häßler
Deutsche Gesellschaft für Suchtforschung und Suchttherapie	Dr. med. Regina Rasenack
Deutsche Gesellschaft für Suchtpsychologie	Prof. Dr. Dipl.-Psych. Tanja Hoff
Deutsche Gesellschaft für Suchtmedizin	PD Dr. med. Gerhard Reymann
Deutsche Gesellschaft für Hebammenwissenschaft	Prof. Dr. rer. medic. Rainhild Schäfers
Deutscher Hebammenverband	Regine Gresens
Berufsverband der deutschen Psychologinnen und Psychologen	Dipl.-Psych. Laszlo A. Pota
Berufsverband der Kinder- und Jugendärzte	Dr. Dr. med. Nikolaus Weissenrieder
Bundesverband der Ärztinnen und Ärzte des Öffentlichen Gesundheitsdienstes	Dr. med. Gabriele Trost-Brinkhues

Tab. 2.2: Am Leitlinienprojekt beteiligte Expertinnen und Experten

Expertinnen/Experten	Funktion
Dipl.-Psych. Gela Becker	Fachliche Leiterin Evangelisches Kinderheim Sonnenhof
Dr. med. Beate Erbas	Bayerische Akademie für Sucht- und Gesundheitsfragen
Dr. Dipl.-Psych. Reinhold Feldmann	FASD-Zentrum Universität Münster
PD Dr. med. Anne Hilgendorff	Neonatologie und Neuropädiatrie, Universität München (LMU)
Dr. med. Heike Hoff-Emden	Chefärztin KMG Rehabilitationszentrum Sülzhayn
Dr. med. Ulrike Horacek	Vorstandsmitglied der DGSPJ, Gesundheitsamt Recklinghausen
Prof. Dr. med. Ina Kopp	Leiterin AWMF-IMWi (nicht stimmberechtigt)
Dr. med. Dipl.-Psych. Mirjam N. Landgraf	Neuropädiatrie, FASD-Ambulanz, iSPZ, Universität München (LMU)
Gisela Michalowski	Vorsitzende der Patientenvertretung FASD Deutschland e. V.
Veerle Moubax	Vorstand der Patientenvertretung FASD Deutschland e. V.
Dr. med. Monika Nothacker	ÄZQ (nicht stimmberechtigt)
Carla Pertl	Stadtjugendamt München

Expertinnen/Experten	Funktion
Dr. Eva Rehfueß	IBE, Universität München (LMU; nicht stimmberechtigt)
Dr. med. Monika Reincke	Referat für Gesundheit und Umwelt der Landeshauptstadt München, Gesundheitsvorsorge für Kinder und Jugendliche
Andreas Rösslein	Neonatologie, Universität München (LMU)
Gila Schindler	Rechtsanwältin für Kinder- und Jugendhilferecht
Prof. Dr. med. Andreas Schulze	Leiter der Neonatologie, Universität München (LMU)
Dr. med. Martin Sobanski	Kinder- und Jugendpsychiatrie, FASD-Ambulanz, Heckscher Klinikum, München
Prof. Dr. med. Hans-Ludwig Spohr	FASD-Zentrum, Charité Berlin
Dipl.-Psych. Penelope Thomas	Kinder- und Jugendpsychiatrie, FASD-Ambulanz, Heckscher Klinikum, München
Dipl.-Psych. Jessica Wagner	FASD-Zentrum, Charité Berlin
Dr. med. Wendelina Wendenburg	Vorstand der Patientenvertretung FASD Deutschland e. V.

2.2 Literaturrecherche und Evidenzbewertung

Die Literaturrecherche wurde in zwei Bereiche eingeteilt, die fokussierte und die systematische Literaturrecherche.

Die fokussierte Literaturrecherche befasste sich mit Hintergrundinformationen, die die Leitliniengruppe relevant für die Ziele der Sensibilisierung des Helfer- und Gesundheitssystems und der Aufklärung der Gesellschaft hielt.

Diese Hintergrundinformationen beinhalten:

- Prävalenz von mütterlichem Alkoholkonsum in der Schwangerschaft und Prävalenz des FAS (Recherche durch Peer Voss und Dr. Eva Rehfueß, Institut für Medizinische Informationsverarbeitung, Biometrie und Epidemiologie, LMU München)
- Risikofaktoren für mütterlichen Alkoholkonsum während der Schwangerschaft (Recherche durch Dr. med. Dipl.-Psych. Mirjam N. Landgraf, Leitlinienkoordinatorin, Abteilung für Pädiatrische Neurologie, Entwicklungsneurologie und Sozialpädiatrie, LMU München)
- Risikofaktoren für die Entwicklung eines FAS (Recherche durch PD Dr. med. Anne Hilgendorff, Abteilung für Pädiatrische Neurologie, Entwicklungsneurologie und Sozialpädiatrie sowie Abteilung für Neonatologie, LMU München)

Die methodische Strategie der fokussierten Literaturrecherche ist aus ▶ Anhang 1 ersichtlich.

Den anderen Teilbereich der Literaturrecherche stellte die systematische Literaturrecherche über diagnostische Kriterien des FAS und deren Evidenzbewertung dar und wurde von Fr. Dr. Monika Nothacker vom Ärztlichen Zentrum für Qualität in der Medizin (ÄZQ) in intensiver dialogischer Rücksprache und Korrektur durch die Leitlinienkoordinatorin Fr. Dr. med. Dipl.-Psych. Mirjam N. Landgraf durchgeführt.

Die Schlüsselfrage der systematischen Literaturrecherche wurde in der ersten Konsensuskonferenz am 14. 09. 2011 im Bundesministerium für Gesundheit in Bonn folgendermaßen konsentiert: Welche Kriterien ermöglichen entwicklungsbezogen die Diagnose eines Fetalen Alkoholsyndroms (FAS) im Kindes- und Jugendalter (0–18 Jahre)?

Die diagnostischen Kriterien für das FAS wurden, orientiert an den bisherigen internationalen Leitlinien, durch die Leitliniengruppe in die vier diagnostische Säulen (1) Wachstumsauffälligkeiten, (2) Faciale Auffälligkeiten, (3) ZNS-Auffälligkeiten und (4) Alkoholkonsum der Mutter während der Schwangerschaft unterteilt.

Zu den vier Diagnose-Säulen wurden folgende Fragen an die systematische Literaturrecherche gestellt und konsentiert:

(1) Prä- und/oder postnatale Wachstumsstörung
Welche Art der Wachstumsstörung im Hinblick auf Gewichts-, Längen- und Kopfumfangsmaße im Alter von 0–18 Jahren ist mit der Diagnose FAS assoziiert?

(2) Faciale Auffälligkeiten
Welche facialen Auffälligkeiten oder Kombinationen davon treten beim FAS im Alter von 0–18 Jahren auf (basierend auf den vorliegenden internationalen Leitlinien: 1. kurze Lidachsen, 2. schmales Oberlippenrot, 3. verstrichenes Philtrum)?

(3) ZNS-Auffälligkeiten
Welche cerebralen Störungen (funktionell und/oder strukturell) sind im Alter zwischen 0 und 18 Jahren mit der Diagnose FAS assoziiert und welche Teilbereiche funktioneller Störungen sind bei Kindern mit FAS typischerweise betroffen?

(4) Alkoholkonsum der Mutter während der Schwangerschaft
Welche Gewichtung hat die Bestätigung des mütterlichen Alkoholkonsums in der Schwangerschaft für die Diagnose eines FAS bei Kindern und Jugendlichen (0–18 Jahre)?

Als Outcome-Kriterien wurden konsentiert:

- Konzeptualisierung der Betreuungsaufgabe durch die richtige Diagnose zum frühestmöglichen Zeitpunkt
- Vermeidung von Fehlbehandlung
- Verbesserung des Funktionsniveaus/der Teilhabe

- Reduktion von:
  - psychiatrischen Erkrankungen
  - Schulversagen und -abbruch (bzw. höhere Rate an Schulabschlüssen und Berufsausbildungen)
  - Delinquenz
  - Misshandlung
  - Krankenhaus- oder sonstigen stationären Aufenthalten
- Entlastung der Eltern (biologische, Pflege- und Adoptiv-Eltern) und Verbesserung der Lebensqualität der gesamten betroffenen Familie
- Verbesserung der sozialen Kompetenz, Ausbau des Freundeskreises, Stabilisierung des Umfelds
- Stärkung der Rolle der Väter als hilfreiche Unterstützer einer alkoholfreien Schwangerschaft
- Reduktion von mütterlichem Alkoholkonsum in den Folge-Schwangerschaften
- Aufklärung der Gesellschaft über die lebenslangen negativen Folgen von intrauteriner Alkoholexposition
- Langfristig Reduktion der Inzidenz von FAS durch Aufklärung

Als Confounder in der Literaturbewertung wurden konsentiert:

1. Normwerte der facialen Auffälligkeiten in den verschiedenen Altersgruppen
2. Intelligenz.

Folgende internationale diagnostische Leitlinien zum FAS wurden in der Literaturrecherche über die letzten 10 Jahre gefunden und bei der Entwicklung handlungsleitender Empfehlungen für die Diagnose FAS in Deutschland berücksichtigt (das methodische Prozedere ist im Leitlinienbericht dargestellt):

1. Astley S (2004) Diagnostic Guide for Fetal Alcohol Spectrum Disorders: The 4-Digit Diagnostic Code. University of Washington Publication Services.
2. National Centre on Birth Defects and Developmental Disabilities (2004) Fetal Alcohol Syndrome: Guidelines for Referral and Diagnosis. Centre for Disease Control.
3. Hoyme HE et al. (2005) A practical clinical approach to diagnosis of fetal alcohol spectrum disorders: Clarification of the 1996 Institute of Medicine Criteria. Paediatrics 115:47.
4. Chudley A et al. (2005) Fetal alcohol spectrum disorder: Canadian guidelines for diagnosis. Can Med Assoc J 172.

Keine dieser internationalen Leitlinien erfüllt nach den AWMF-Vorgaben die methodischen Kriterien einer S3-Leitlinie.

Die systematische Literaturrecherche erfolgte gemäß der im Leitlinienbericht und in ▶ Anhang 2 dargestellten Strategie. Die Recherche umfasste englisch- und deutschsprachige Literatur im Zeitraum von 01.01.2001 bis 31.10.2011. Nach Sichtung der Abstracts und der daraus ausgewählten

Volltexte wurden insgesamt 178 Publikationen zur Evidenzbewertung eingeschlossen (▶ Abb. 2.2).

Die vom ÄZQ während der systematischen Literaturrecherche nicht beschaffbare Publikation konnte von den Leitlinienkoordinatoren nach Abschluss des Evidenzberichtes beschafft werden. Aus der Publikation Roussotte et al. (2011, Abnormal brain activation during working memory in children with prenatal exposure to drugs of abuse: The effects of methamphetamine, alcohol, and polydrug exposure. NeuroImage 54:3067–3075) resultierte keine inhaltliche Änderung der Leitlinie.

Die resultierenden Volltexte über diagnostische Kriterien des FAS wurden, soweit möglich, mit dem Oxford-Evidenzklassifikations-System für diagnostische Studien (2009) bewertet (siehe Leitlinienbericht).

Kohortenstudien wurden entsprechend der Oxford-Evidenzklassifikation in explorative Kohortenstudien mit einem Level of Evidence von 2 b (LoE 2 b) und Validierungskohortenstudien mit einem LoE 1 b unterteilt. Bei einer Validierungskohortenstudie wird ein, in einer explorativen Studie identifiziertes, diagnostisches Merkmal an einem unabhängigen Kollektiv überprüft. Nicht-konsekutive Kohortenstudien oder solche mit sehr kleiner Teilnehmerzahl wurden mit einem LoE von 3 b, Fall-Kontroll-Studien mit einem LoE von 4 bewertet.

Lediglich ein Review der systematischen Literaturrecherche kann als systematischer Review von guter methodischer Qualität über einen Zeitraum bis Juli 2008 bezeichnet werden (mit Evidenzklassifikation des NHMRC): Elliott et al. (2008) [31] Fetal Alcohol Spectrum Disorders (FASD): systematic reviews of prevention, diagnosis and management.

Bei den übrigen Reviews mit Angabe einer systematischen Recherche fehlen meist Suchfragen, Angaben zu Treffern, Ein- und Ausschlusskriterien sowie eine Beschreibung oder Bewertung der methodischen Güte der eingeschlossenen Studien. Die Studienqualität für diese Reviews ist als mäßig bis schlecht zu bezeichnen. Aus diesen Reviews kann ein inhaltlicher Überblick der beschriebenen Ergebnisse gegeben werden, eine Beurteilung der Qualität der zugrundeliegenden Studien ist nicht durchgehend möglich.

Die Literaturliste der eingeschlossenen Studien bei der systematischen Literaturrecherche befindet sich in ▶ Anhang 5.

Die Zuverlässigkeit der Aussagen, die auf Studien mit bekannten Fällen (Kinder mit der Diagnose FAS) und Kontrollen (gesunde Kinder) basieren, ist begrenzt, da die Diagnosen bereits feststehen. Häufig fällt auch eine hohe Prävalenzrate von Kindern mit FAS in den Studienpopulationen auf, die die Übertragung der Studienergebnisse auf eine Normalpopulation problematisch macht. Diagnostische Studien zum Fetalen Alkoholsyndrom stellen bezüglich eines optimalen Studiendesigns eine besondere Herausforderung dar. Für gute diagnostische Studien ist allgemein ein unabhängiger verlässlicher Referenzstandard erforderlich. Die Validierung von diagnostischen FAS-Kriterien wurde jedoch an bereits mit FAS diagnostizierten Kindern und Jugendlichen

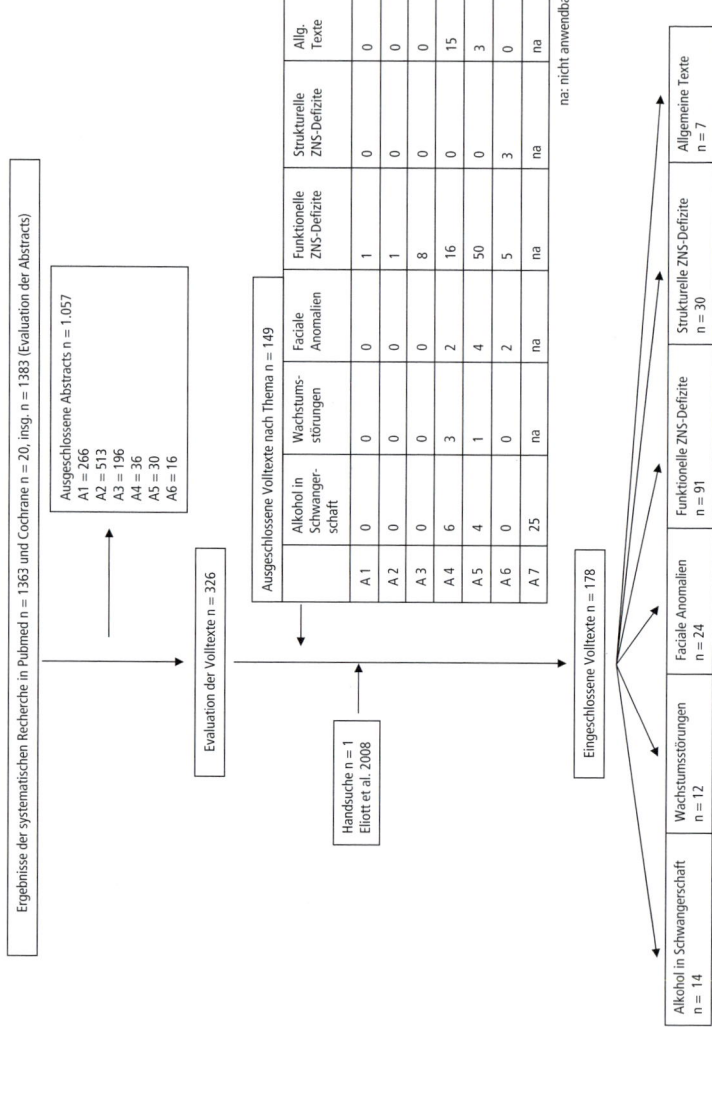

Abb. 2.2: Ablauf der systematischen Literaturrecherche

überprüft. Dafür wurden unterschiedliche Instrumente angewendet (vor allem IOM-Kriterien und 4-Digit Diagnostic Code), die aufgrund der differenten diagnostischen Kriterien oder Cut-off-Werte (Perzentile von Kopfumfangskurven, Anzahl facialer Auffälligkeiten, Berücksichtigung funktioneller ZNS-Auffälligkeiten) in ihrer diagnostischen Diskrimination nicht übereinstimmen. Insbesondere die facialen Kriterien unterliegen einem sogenannten Incorporation-Bias, bei dem das Testkriterium grundsätzlich auch Teil des Referenzstandards ist. In den meisten Studien wurden als Vergleichsgruppen Kinder und Jugendliche gewählt, deren Mütter keinen Alkoholkonsum während der Schwangerschaft angaben. Dabei sollte allerdings berücksichtigt werden, dass die Aussagen zum mütterlichen Alkoholkonsum in der Schwangerschaft wahrscheinlich häufig aufgrund sozialer Erwünschtheit ungenau und retrospektiv auch nicht objektivierbar sind. Daher könnten sich auch in den gesunden Kontrollgruppen Kinder mit intrauteriner Alkoholexposition befinden und den Vergleich mit Kindern mit FAS beeinträchtigen.

2.3 Erstellung von Evidenztabellen

Die vom Ärztlichen Zentrum für Qualität in der Medizin erstellten Evidenztabellen der Literatur über diagnostische Kriterien des FAS sind in ▶ Anhang 4 dargestellt.

2.4 Formale Konsensfindung und Formulierung von Empfehlungen

Anhand der evidenzbewerteten Studien wurden von den Leitlinienkoordinatoren Empfehlungsvorschläge für die Diagnostik des FAS erarbeitet. Diese Empfehlungen wurden in der zweiten (17.02.12) und dritten (25.05.12) Konsensuskonferenz von der Leitliniengruppe diskutiert, je nach klinischer Relevanz modifiziert und graduiert. Die daraus resultierenden handlungsleitenden Empfehlungen für die Diagnostik des FAS bei Kindern und Jugendlichen in Deutschland wurden in den gleichen Konsensussitzungen mittels einer formalen Konsensfindung in Form eines nominalen Gruppenprozesses konsentiert.

Der nominale Gruppenprozess wurde in den folgenden Schritten unter Moderation von Fr. Prof. Ina Kopp (AWMF) durchgeführt:

1. Präsentation der Ergebnisse der Literaturrecherche und der darauf basierenden, zu konsentierenden Leitlinien-Empfehlungen

2. Verfassen von Änderungsvorschlägen und Anmerkungen zu den vorgeschlagenen diagnostischen Kriterien und Empfehlungen durch jeden Teilnehmer der Konsensuskonferenz
3. Die Änderungsvorschläge wurden der Reihe nach von Fr. Prof. Kopp als unabhängiger und nicht stimmberechtigter Moderatorin abgefragt, schriftlich festgehalten und per Beamer für alle sichtbar projiziert.
4. Vorhergehende Abstimmung aller diagnostischen Kriterien, Empfehlungen und Empfehlungsgrade sowie der Änderungsvorschläge
5. Diskussion der Punkte, für die kein Konsens erzielt werden konnte
6. Endgültige Abstimmung und Protokollierung der Konsensstärke.

Alle Empfehlungen, bis auf die Cut-off-Perzentilenkurve des Kopfumfangs, wurden im „starken Konsens" (Zustimmung von > 95 % der Teilnehmer) oder im Konsens (Zustimmung von > 75 % der Teilnehmer) verabschiedet.

Die Abstimmungs- und Ergebnisprotokolle der Sitzungen können über die Leitlinienkoordinatorin angefordert und eingesehen werden.

Bei den Empfehlungen wurde zwischen drei Empfehlungsgraden unterschieden, deren unterschiedliche Qualität durch die Formulierung („soll", „sollte", „kann") ausgedrückt wird. In der Regel bestimmt die Evidenzstärke den Empfehlungsgrad (▶ Abb. 2.3):

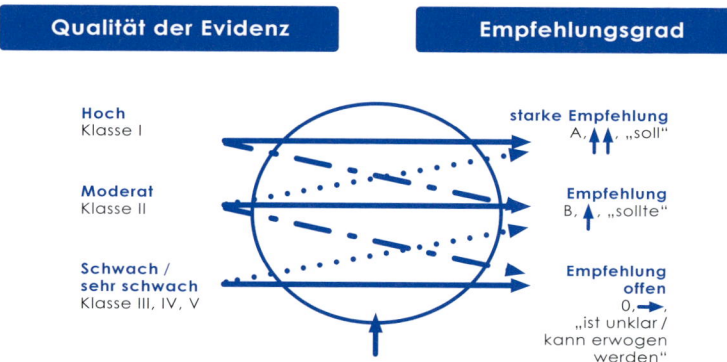

Abb. 2.3: Bestimmung von Empfehlungsgraden anhand der Evidenzbewertung der Literatur (mit Genehmigung von Fr. Prof. Kopp, AWMF)

In der 2. und 3. Konsensuskonferenz wurden die Ergebnisse der Literatur mit den jeweils bestimmten Evidenzklassen präsentiert und die von den Leitlinienkoordinatoren vorgeschlagenen diagnostischen Kriterien und Empfehlungen inklusive der Empfehlungsgrade durch die Leitliniengruppe diskutiert. Bei der Festlegung der endgültigen Empfehlungsgrade im formalen Konsensusverfahren durch die Leitliniengruppe wurden neben der zugrundeliegenden Evidenzstärke auch die methodische Qualität der gesamten bisherigen Literatur zum Thema FAS, die klinische Relevanz der Studien, die Umsetzbarkeit in die Praxis und ethische Verpflichtungen berücksichtigt.

2.5 Verabschiedung

Die Mandatsträgerinnen und -träger der deutschen Fachgesellschaften und Berufsverbände sowie die Expertinnen und Experten der Konsensusgruppe hatten die Möglichkeit, Anmerkungen oder Korrekturen zum Leitlinienbericht und zur Leitlinie zu machen. Anhand dieser Anregungen wurde die Leitlinie von der Leitlinienkoordinatorin Fr. Dr. med. Dipl.-Psych. Mirjam N. Landgraf modifiziert. Die Mandatsträger mit der vollen Prokura ihrer Fachgesellschaft stimmten den Inhalten der Leitlinie eigenständig zu. Andere Mandatsträger präsentierten die Leitlinie den Vorständen oder Leitliniengremien ihrer Fachgesellschaften oder Berufsverbände. Diese stimmten nach kleinen redaktionellen Änderungen (keine konsenspflichtigen inhaltlichen Anpassungen) der Leitlinie zu und erreichten damit die Verabschiedung der Leitlinie.

2.6 Verbreitung und Implementierung

Die Kurz- und Langfassung der Leitlinie sowie der Leitlinienbericht sind auf der Homepage der AWMF (www.amwf.org) veröffentlicht, um deren Inhalte allen Interessierten frei zugänglich zu machen.

Zur Implementierung der empfohlenen diagnostischen Kriterien wurde ein Pocket Guide für alle Beteiligten des Gesundheits- und Hilfesystems entworfen. Dieser Pocket Guide (▶ Pocket Guide am Buchanfang) beinhaltet den Algorithmus für die Abklärung des Fetalen Alkoholsyndroms bei Kindern und Jugendlichen sowie die konsentierten diagnostischen Kriterien in Gegenüberstellung zu möglichen Differentialdiagnosen des FAS in der jeweiligen diagnostischen Säule. Web-Adressen mit Links zu weiterführenden Informationen über das Krankheitsbild FAS, zur vorliegenden Leitlinie und zur Homepage der Patientenvertretung FASD Deutschland e. V. befinden sich ebenfalls im Pocket Guide.

Bei Formulierung eines Verdachtes auf FAS oder bei Unsicherheit hinsichtlich der Diagnose FAS soll der betreuende professionelle Helfer, einschließlich Pflegepersonal, Hebammen, Geburtshelfer, Psychologen, Sozialpädagogen, Sozialarbeiter, Therapeuten, klinisch oder institutionell tätige oder niedergelassene Ärzte der Gynäkologie, der Kinder- und Jugendmedizin einschließlich der Schwerpunktgebiete Neonatologie, Intensivmedizin, Neuropädiatrie, der Kinder- und Jugendpsychiatrie, Psychotherapie und Psychosomatik, der Allgemeinmedizin und des öffentlichen Gesundheitsdienstes, das Kind zur weiterführenden Diagnostik an einen FAS-erfahrenen Leistungserbringer überweisen. Der Algorithmus veranschaulicht die für diese Leitlinie konsentierten Kriterien, anhand derer die Diagnose eines FAS in Deutschland gestellt werden soll.

Ein Ziel der Leitliniengruppe ist die Sensibilisierung des Helfer- und Gesundheitssystems gegenüber Alkoholkonsum in der Schwangerschaft mit seinen schwerwiegenden und lebenslangen Folgen und gegenüber dem Krankheitsbild FAS mithilfe der vorliegenden Leitlinie. In den Konsensuskonferenzen wurde diskutiert, dass der Verdacht auf ein FAS vermehrt gestellt werden soll und die betroffenen Kinder baldmöglichst zu Experten geschickt werden sollen, die sich intensiv mit dem Krankheitsbild FAS auseinandersetzen und entsprechende Kompetenzen personell und institutionell vorhalten. Laut den statistischen Schätzungen über die Prävalenz des FAS aus den USA, Kanada und Europa bekommen viel zu wenige Kinder mit FAS in Deutschland tatsächlich auch die Diagnose FAS. Das Erhalten der Diagnose FAS ist jedoch unabdingbar für eine adäquate Förderung, Beschulung, Ausbildung und Unterbringung des Kindes oder Jugendlichen mit FAS sowie zur Reduktion von Sekundärerkrankungen. Außerdem kann erst durch die richtige Diagnose eine individuelle Unterstützung und Entlastung der betroffenen Familie erreicht werden.

Da aktuell noch zu wenige auf FAS spezialisierte Anlaufstellen in Deutschland existieren, ist es dringend notwendig, Fortbildungen für die verschiedenen involvierten Berufsgruppen zu halten. Die Leitliniengruppe legt sich dabei nicht nur auf die Ärzteschaft oder die Psychologen als Experten fest, sondern hofft, auch bei anderen Berufsgruppen für das Thema FAS Interesse und Aufmerksamkeit zu wecken. Die Diagnose FAS sollte bei Kindern und Jugendlichen interdisziplinär gestellt werden, wobei die abschließende ärztliche und psychologische Beurteilung einen besonders hohen Stellenwert hat.

Die Mandatsträger der beteiligten Fachgesellschaften werden versuchen, in ihrem Fachbereich das Krankheitsbild FAS intensiv zu kommunizieren und über dessen Symptome und Komplikationen im Rahmen von Kongressen oder Fortbildungen aufzuklären.

Die Gesellschaft für Neuropädiatrie als federführende Gesellschaft der vorliegenden Leitlinie hat als ihre Verantwortliche für FASD die Leitlinienkoordinatorin Fr. Dr. med. Dipl.-Psych. Mirjam N. Landgraf bestimmt. Im Rahmen der Jahrestagung der Gesellschaft für Neuropädiatrie wird jährlich ein Treffen der FASD-Experten und FASD-Interessierten unter Leitung von Fr. Dr. med. Dipl.-Psych. Mirjam N. Landgraf stattfinden.

2.7 Finanzierung der Leitlinie und Darlegung möglicher Interessenkonflikte

Die Entwicklung der Leitlinie wurde durch die Drogenbeauftragte der Bundesregierung, Fr. Dr. Dyckmans, initiiert und im Wesentlichen durch das Bundesministerium für Gesundheit finanziert. Personalkosten für die Leitlinienkoordinatorin und eine wissenschaftliche Hilfskraft, Kosten für die Aufträge an das IBE München, an das Ärztliche Zentrum für Qualität in der Medizin (ÄZQ) und an ein Design-Büro sowie Reisekosten und Sachkosten wurden vom Bundesministerium für Gesundheit für 18 Monate übernommen. Die überwiegende Finanzierung der Leitlinie durch das Bundesministerium für Gesundheit hat zu keinen inhaltlichen Interferenzen oder Anpassungen der Leitlinie geführt. Die Gesellschaft für Neuropädiatrie und der Landesverband Bayern für körper- und mehrfachbehinderte Menschen e. V. als Träger des iSPZ München haben das Projekt zusätzlich unterstützt. Weitere Kosten wurden durch das Dr. von Haunersche Kinderspital des Universitätsklinikums München LMU getragen.

Alle Mitglieder der Münchner Steuergruppe und der deutschlandweiten Konsensusgruppe legten eventuelle Interessenkonflikte schriftlich offen. Die Interessenkonflikterklärungen wurden bei der Leitlinienkoordinatorin gesammelt und sind zusammengefasst im Leitlinienbericht dargestellt (http://www.awmf.org/leitlinien/detail/ll/022-025.html).

Alle Konsensusmitglieder gaben an, sich keinerlei finanzielle, berufliche oder persönliche Vorteile durch die Inhalte der Leitlinie zu versprechen.

2.8 Gültigkeitsdauer und Aktualisierungsverfahren

Die Gültigkeit der Leitlinie ist auf fünf Jahre festgelegt. Um die Aktualität der Leitlinie zu gewährleisten, wird in einer jährlichen Umfrage durch die Leitlinienkoordinatoren unter den Mandatsträgern, Experten und Patientenvertretern geklärt, ob dringende Gründe für eine vorzeitige Aktualisierung der Leitlinie vorliegen. Falls vorzeitige Aktualisierungen der Leitlinie erfolgen, werden diese in einem Addendum auf der Website der AWMF und der Gesellschaft für Neuropädiatrie (als die, durch die Deutsche Gesellschaft für Kinder- und Jugendmedizin DGKJ zur Federführung ernannte, Gesellschaft) publiziert.

3 Hintergrundinformationen: Ergebnisse der fokussierten Literaturrecherche

3.1 Prävalenz von mütterlichem Alkoholkonsum in der Schwangerschaft und Prävalenz des Fetalen Alkoholsyndroms

Insgesamt beschäftigten sich in den letzten zehn Jahren 17 Studien mit der Prävalenz von mütterlichem Alkoholkonsum während der Schwangerschaft und 13 Studien mit FAS-Prävalenzen und FAS-Inzidenzen.

Der methodische Prozess und die Literaturliste dieses Teilbereiches der fokussierten Literaturrecherche sind ▶ Anhang 1 zu entnehmen.

3.1.1 Europa

Für den Kontinent Europa erfüllten insgesamt zehn Studien die Einschlusskriterien, darunter jeweils zwei Studien aus Italien und Norwegen und jeweils eine Studie aus Schweden, Deutschland, Frankreich, Dänemark, England und Irland.

Alkoholkonsum während der Schwangerschaft

Mit der Häufigkeit von Alkoholkonsum in der Schwangerschaft haben sich insgesamt neun Studien in Italien (May et al. 2006; May et al. 2011), Frankreich (de Chazeron et al. 2011), Schweden (Goransson et al. 2003), Norwegen (Elgen et al. 2007; Alvik et al. 2006), Irland (Donnelly et al. 2008), Dänemark (Strandberg-Larsen et al. 2008) und Deutschland (Bergmann et al. 2007) beschäftigt. Die Daten beziehen sich auf den Zeitraum von 2000 bis 2008 und umfassen mehr als 108 000 Mütter. Die beobachteten Werte bewegen sich zwischen 10,8 % und 91,7 %. Laut KIGGS-Studie des Robert Koch-Instituts zur Gesundheit von Kindern und Jugendlichen betrug in Deutschland der Alkoholkonsum während der Schwangerschaft von Müttern der eingeschlossenen Kinder 14,4 % und stieg bis 2005 auf 16,2 %. Allerdings verwenden diese Studien sehr unterschiedliche Definitionen bezüglich Häufigkeit, Zeitpunkt und Ausmaß des Alkoholkonsums. Werden jedoch der Alkoholkonsum vor dem Bekanntwerden der Schwangerschaft oder der einmalige geringe Alkoholkonsum während der Schwangerschaft ausgeschlossen und werden kleinere und deshalb weniger zuverlässige Studien ebenfalls nicht berücksichtigt, so ergibt sich eine Bandbreite von 14,4 % bis 30,0 %. Konzentriert man sich auf den Teilaspekt des sogenannten „binge drinking" (exzessiver Alkoholkonsum zu einer Gelegenheit, „Sturz-Trinken", „Komasaufen") bewegen sich die Prävalenz-Zahlen zwischen 1,2 % und 3,5 %. Dabei ist zu beachten, dass Schwangere, die nur zu einer Gelegenheit exzessiv Alkohol getrunken hatten (binge drinking) und zu diesem Zeitpunkt nicht gewusst hatten, dass sie schwanger sind, nicht mit einbezogen wurden. Die Prävalenz-Zahlen könnten in Wirklichkeit aufgrund der Dunkelziffer wesentlich höher ausfallen, da Mütter aus Angst vor sozialer Stigmatisierung wahrscheinlich häufig falsche (alkoholverneinende) Angaben zu ihrem Alkoholkonsum machen.

Prävalenz des Fetalen Alkoholsyndroms

Mit FAS-Prävalenzen haben sich vier Studien aus Italien (May et al. 2006; May et al. 2011), England (Morleo et al. 2011) und Frankreich (de Chazeron et al. 2011) beschäftigt. Die Daten beziehen sich auf die Jahre 1997 bis 2008 und umfassen insgesamt 2840 Kinder. Die Prävalenzen von FAS bewegen sich zwischen 0,2 und 8,2 pro 1000 Geburten. Kritisch zu betrachten ist die Studie aus England, die zu einem Ergebnis von 0,8 pro 100 000 Geburten kam. Diese Prävalenz ist im Vergleich zu den anderen Studien auffallend niedrig.

Verglichen mit anderen neuropädiatrischen Erkrankungen wie dem Down-Syndrom mit einer Prävalenz von ca. 0,1–0,2 % (Loane et al. Twenty-year trends in the prevalence of Down syndrome and other trisomies in Europe: impact of maternal age and prenatal screening. European Journal of Human Genetics 2012) und der Cerebralparese mit einer Prävalenz von ca. 0,2–0,3 % (Heinen et al. The updated European Consensus 2009 on the use of Botulinum toxin for children with cerebral palsy. European Journal of Paediatric Neurology 2010; 14:45–66) ist das Fetale Alkoholsyndrom in Deutschland sehr häufig. Allerdings wird die Diagnose FAS viel zu selten gestellt, da die professionellen Helfer im Gesundheitssystem Hemmungen haben, einen diesbezüglichen Verdacht auszusprechen oder zu wenig über das Krankheitsbild informiert sind.

Das Vollbild des Fetalen Alkoholsyndroms tritt nach Expertenschätzung nur bei einem kleinen Prozentsatz aller Kinder mit pränatalen Alkohol-Folgeschäden auf. Das bedeutet, dass die Fetale Alkoholspektrumstörung eine der häufigsten angeborenen Erkrankungen darstellt, ohne als solche bislang erkannt und berücksichtigt zu werden.

Alkoholkonsum während der Schwangerschaft ist dabei eine der ganz wenigen vollständig vermeidbaren Ursachen für schwere Entwicklungsstörungen beim Kind.

3.1.2 USA

Mit FAS-Prävalenzen und den Häufigkeiten von Alkoholkonsum in der Schwangerschaft beschäftigten sich 15 Studien aus den Vereinigten Staaten von Amerika.

Alkoholkonsum während der Schwangerschaft

Insgesamt beschäftigen sich acht Studien in 50 Staaten der USA mit dem Alkoholkonsum von Schwangeren (Centres for Disease Control and Prevention 2009; Aliyu et al. 2009; Tsai et al. 2007; Chambers et al. 2005; Drews et al. 2003; O'Connor et al. 2003; Ethen et al. 2009; Grant et al. 2009). Die Daten beziehen sich auf den Zeitraum von 1989 bis 2004 und mehr als 430 000 Mütter wurden befragt. In USA beläuft sich die Häufigkeit auf 8,0–30,0 % für jeglichen Alkoholkonsum. Für das binge drinking ergab sich eine Prävalenz von 1,0–8,3 %. Hier ist zu bedenken, dass einige Studien sich auf bestimmte Ethnizitäten wie die schwarze, lateinamerikanische oder Inuit-Population der USA beziehen (Chambers et al. 2005; O'Connor et al. 2003). In Zusammenschau aller amerikanischen Studien können wegen der hohen Anzahl der Teilnehmerinnen diese Zahlen trotzdem als repräsentativ für den Alkoholkonsum von Schwangeren in den USA angesehen werden.

Prävalenz des FAS

Acht Studien, die fast sämtliche Staaten der USA abdecken, machen Angaben zu FAS-Prävalenzen (Druschel et al. 2007; Astley 2004; Weiss et al. 2004; Fox et al. 2003; Poitra et al. 2003; Centres for Disease Control and Prevention 2002; Astley et al. 2002; U. S. Government 2003). Die Daten beziehen sich auf den Zeitraum von 1992 bis 2004 und umfassen insgesamt fast eine halbe Million Kinder. Die Studien kommen zu einer Prävalenz-Bandbreite von 0,2–4,5 pro 1000 Geburten. Hier ist aufgrund ihrer guten Datenlage für 35 Bundesstaaten, basierend auf Birth-Defects-Surveillance-Daten, insbesondere die Studie der US-Regierung von 2003 hervorzuheben. Weiterhin ist, wie oben bereits erwähnt, zu beachten, dass sich manche Studien vorwiegend mit bestimmten ethnischen Bevölkerungsgruppen der USA beschäftigt haben; auch hier bewegen sich die Häufigkeiten zwischen 0,2 und 4,5 pro 1000 Geburten.

3.1.3 Kanada

Für Kanada wurde eine Studie gefunden, die sich mit mütterlichem Alkoholkonsum während der Schwangerschaft befasste. Die Studie ermittelte einen Alkoholkonsum während der Schwangerschaft von 5,4 % für Ontario und

7,2 % für British Columbia (Thanh et al. 2010). Außerdem extrapolierten die Autoren die Ergebnisse und schätzten für ganz Kanada einen mütterlichen Alkoholkonsum von 5,8 %. Diese Daten basieren auf dem auf nationaler und Provinzebene repräsentativen Canadian Community Health Survey. Das Wahlmodul zu Alkoholkonsum während der Schwangerschaft wurde allerdings nur in zwei Provinzen umgesetzt, so dass die Zahlen für ganz Kanada kritisch zu betrachten sind. Studien zur Häufigkeit von FAS konnten unter Berücksichtigung der Einschlusskriterien nicht gefunden werden.

3.1.4 Anmerkungen zur Qualität der Studien

Die 27 eingeschlossenen Studien zeichnen sich durch große Heterogenität in Studiendesign, Auswahl und Anzahl der Teilnehmerinnen und Teilnehmer sowie in verwendeten Definitionen aus.

Ein Großteil der Studien sind Querschnittsstudien, andere beziehen sich auf Vitalstatistiken z. B. Aliyu et al. 2009) oder Register (z. B. Fox et al. 2003) oder wurden als integrierter Bestandteil groß angelegter Kohortenstudien durchgeführt (z. B. Bergmann et al. 2007). Studien zum Alkoholkonsum während der Schwangerschaft setzen bezüglich der untersuchten Bevölkerungsgruppe unterschiedliche Schwerpunkte, z. B. bei erstmals schwangeren Frauen (z. B. Donnelly et al. 2008), Frauen, die vor kurzem entbunden haben, (z. B. de Chazeron et al. 2011) oder Müttern von Kleinkindern (z. B. Thanh et al. 2010). Auch bezüglich der Häufigkeit von FAS unterscheiden sich die betrachteten Bevölkerungsgruppen erheblich; so werden Daten zur Prävalenz für Neugeborene, Kinder im Grundschulalter und Jugendliche, für unterschiedliche Ethnien sowie für adoptierte oder Pflegekinder (z. B. Astley et al. 2002) erhoben. Die Auswahl der betrachteten Bevölkerungsgruppe kann erhebliche Auswirkungen auf die Wahrscheinlichkeit von Recall Bias (Frauen, bei denen eine Schwangerschaft schon Jahre zurückliegt, erinnern sich weniger genau an ihren Alkoholkonsum als aktuell schwangere Frauen), Social Desirability Bias (Frauen, für deren Kind eine FAS-Diagnose vorliegt, neigen eher dazu, einen Alkoholkonsum zu verschweigen, als Frauen gesunder Kinder) und andere systematische Verzerrungen haben. Auch wenn die Studienqualität nicht systematisch bewertet wurde, ist anzumerken, dass sich die Studien hinsichtlich der Auswahl der Studienpopulation (z. B. über Krankenhäuser versus über national repräsentative Studien) und der Anzahl der Studienteilnehmer (sehr kleine Studien mit unter 200 Teilnehmern bis hin zu mehreren Hunderttausend Teilnehmern) erheblich unterscheiden.

Den hier berichteten Zahlen liegen außerdem unterschiedliche Definitionen für den Alkoholkonsum während der Schwangerschaft und für die Diagnose FAS zugrunde. Insbesondere die korrekte Erfassung leichter und mittelschwerer Ausprägungsformen alkoholinduzierter Schädigungen im Neugeborenen- und Kindesalter stellt eine wichtige Fehlerquelle dar und erklärt sicherlich einen Teil der großen Bandbreite. Darüber hinaus ergeben sich für Studien zu FAS generelle Probleme, insbesondere ist davon auszugehen, dass die Dunkelziffer für beide hier betrachteten Endpunkte hoch ist. Bezüglich des Alkoholkonsums während der Schwangerschaft muss man aufgrund des erheblichen gesellschaftlichen Erwartungsdrucks von einem deutlichen Underreporting ausgehen. Bezüglich der FAS-Prävalenz muss berücksichtigt werden, dass Kinder aus Problemfamilien in den meisten nicht national repräsentativen Studien wahrscheinlich nicht angemessen erfasst sind, was zu einer Unterschätzung der eigentlichen Prävalenz führen könnte.

3.2 Risikofaktoren für mütterlichen Alkoholkonsum in der Schwangerschaft

Die primäre Prävention von FAS beinhaltet die Aufklärung von allen Frauen und Männern im zeugungsfähigen Alter über die potentiell verheerende Wirkung von mütterlichem Alkoholkonsum während der Schwangerschaft auf das ungeborene Kind, der zu lebenslangen Einschränkungen führen kann. Die Bestimmung von Risikopopulationen für Alkoholkonsum in der Schwangerschaft ist wichtig, um den betroffenen Frauen und Männern eine intensivierte Aufklärung bieten zu können und damit die Prävalenz von mütterlichem Alkoholkonsum während der Schwangerschaft in der deutschen Gesellschaft senken zu können.

Das methodische Prozedere und die Literaturliste dieses Teilbereichs der fokussierten Literaturrecherche sind ▶ Anhang 1 zu entnehmen.

Die in der Literatur beschriebenen mütterlichen Risikofaktoren wurden zur übersichtlicheren Darstellung in folgende Bereiche eingeteilt:

- Alter
- Nationalität
- Gesundheitsbezogene Risikofaktoren
- Schwangerschaftsbesonderheiten
- Sozioökonomischer Status
- Soziale Umgebung
- Psychologische Risikofaktoren

Die kanadische Originalliteratur wurde aufgrund der geringen Anzahl von Publikationen mit der amerikanischen Literatur über Risikofaktoren für mütterlichen Alkoholkonsum in der Schwangerschaft zusammengefasst.

3.2.1 Risikofaktoren, für mütterlichen Alkoholkonsum in den USA und Kanada

Literatur: ▶ Anhang 1

Alter

Ältere Schwangere scheinen in den USA und Kanada eher risikobehaftet für Alkoholkonsum zu sein als jüngere Schwangere. Das ältere Alter wird in vielen Studien jedoch nicht exakt anhand der Lebensjahre bestimmt oder unterschiedlich definiert, mit einem Altersrange von über 25 Jahren bis über 35 Jahren.

Nationalität

Bei Untersuchungen in Lebensbereichen, die bezüglich der Nationalität oder Ethnizität repräsentativ für die gesamte amerikanische Gesellschaft sind, zeigt sich, dass kaukasische Amerikanerinnen am häufigsten Alkohol während der Schwangerschaft konsumieren. Afro-Amerikanerinnen und hispanische Amerikanerinnen, die in den USA geboren wurden, haben ein größeres Risiko für Alkoholkonsum in der Schwangerschaft als im Ausland geborene Frauen gleicher Ethnizität. Amerikanerinnen nichtkaukasischer Ethnizität, die seit mehreren Generationen in den USA leben oder besser akkulturiert sind (z. B. zuhause vorwiegend amerikanisch sprechen), weisen ein noch höheres Risiko auf.

In diesem Bereich ist problematisch, dass viele Studien eine sehr selektive Stichprobe untersucht haben, z. B. in Reservaten lebende Native American Indians, Inuit oder Schwarz-Amerikanerinnen aus der untersten sozioökonomischen Schicht, die zur unentgeltlichen Geburt in die Klinik kamen. In diesen Studien wird ein hoher Prozentsatz an Alkohol konsumierenden Schwangeren in Minderheiten angenommen. In Minderheiten, deren Religion Alkohol verbietet, trinken dagegen weniger Frauen Alkohol während der Schwangerschaft. Allerdings muss bei kultureller Inakzeptanz immer von einer Beschönigung der Angaben ausgegangen werden.

Gesundheitsbezogene Risikofaktoren

Bei frühem Beginn von Alkoholkonsum, in einer Publikation beschrieben als Alkoholkonsum vor dem 18. Lebensjahr, in einem anderen Artikel als Alkoholkonsum in den College-Jahren, ist das Risiko höher, in der Schwangerschaft Alkohol zu konsumieren.

Mit steigender Häufigkeit und Höhe des Alkoholkonsums vor der Schwangerschaft steigt auch das Risiko von Alkoholkonsum in der Schwangerschaft.

In mehreren Publikationen werden Items aus Alkohol-Screeningverfahren wie dem TWEAK (Items: Tolerance, Worry, Eye opener, Amnesia, Cut down) von Schwangeren beantwortet und es zeigt sich, dass Schwangere mit hohen Screeningwerten häufiger Alkohol konsumieren.

Frauen mit einer Alkoholabhängigkeit, die definiert wurde als durch Alkohol verursachte gesundheitliche Probleme oder als vorhergehende Behandlung wegen Alkoholproblemen, trinken häufiger Alkohol in der Schwangerschaft.

Frauen, die wegen Drogenkonsums behandelt wurden oder vor oder während der Schwangerschaft Drogen konsumieren, sind eher risikobehaftet für Alkoholkonsum während der Schwangerschaft.

In vielen Publikationen wurde einheitlich gezeigt, dass auch Frauen, die vor oder während der Schwangerschaft Nikotin konsumieren, häufiger während der Schwangerschaft Alkohol trinken.

In zwei Publikationen wurde ein hoher Koffeinkonsum als Risikofaktor für mütterlichen Alkoholkonsum gefunden.

Schwangerschaftsbesonderheiten

Die Anzahl der Schwangerschaften als Risikofaktor für den Alkoholkonsum in der Schwangerschaft wird in der amerikanischen und kanadischen Literatur kontrovers diskutiert (▶ Anhang 1).

In den Publikationen wird dagegen einheitlich als Risikofaktor eine unbeabsichtigte oder ungewollte Schwangerschaft dargestellt.

Frauen, die wenig oder spät präpartale Vorsorge in Anspruch nehmen, sind ebenfalls risikobehafteter.

Jeweils eine Publikation beschreibt folgende Risikofaktoren: vorheriges Frühgeborenes, vorheriger Schwangerschaftsabbruch, vorherige Infertilität.

Sozioökonomischer Status

Hinsichtlich des sozioökonomischen Status sind die Ergebnisse der Literatur kontrovers. Häufig wurden Minderheiten oder Gegenden mit insgesamt niedrigem Sozialstatus untersucht, in denen die Schwangeren mit nochmals vergleichsweise niedrigerem Sozialstatus, Arbeitslosigkeit oder Erhalt öffentlicher Zuwendungen häufiger Alkohol während der Schwangerschaft konsumieren als Frauen mit vergleichsweise höherem (aber immer noch niedrigem) sozioökonomischen Status. Wenn Stichproben evaluiert wurden, die repräsentativ für alle Bevölkerungsschichten sind, zeigt sich jedoch ein höheres Risiko für Alkoholkonsum bei schwangeren Frauen, die eine bessere Bildung, ein höheres Einkommen und keine Arbeitslosigkeit aufweisen.

Soziale Umgebung

In sehr vielen Publikationen wurde der Ehestand bei den Befragungen der Schwangeren ermittelt und es zeigt sich übereinstimmend, dass unverheiratete Schwangere häufiger Alkohol konsumieren. Die Unterscheidung zwischen Frauen, die zwar unverheiratet sind aber in fester Beziehung leben und denen, die unverheiratet aber alleinstehend sind, wurde in den Studien nicht immer gemacht. In einigen Publikationen, die jedoch meist in unterprivilegierten Gegenden durchgeführt wurden, ergab sich, dass ein Mangel an sozialer, emotionaler oder finanzieller Unterstützung ein Risiko für Alkoholkonsum der Schwangeren darstellt.

Alkoholkonsum des Partners oder Alkoholkonsum in der Familie sind weitere Risikofaktoren für mütterlichen Alkoholkonsum. Auch Drogenkonsum des Partners, der Familie oder der Freunde scheinen einen Einfluss auf den Alkoholkonsum der Schwangeren zu haben.

In einzelnen Publikationen wird darauf hingewiesen, dass Frauen, die Verletzungen erlitten, seien sie selbst- oder fremdverursacht sowie unter oder ohne Alkoholeinfluss entstanden, eine Risikopopulation für Alkoholkonsum in der Schwangerschaft darstellen.

In zwei Publikationen wurde evaluiert, dass der seltene oder der fehlende Besuch von religiösen Einrichtungen bzw. Zeremonien ein Risikofaktor für Alkoholkonsum sein kann.

Psychologische Risikofaktoren

Viele Publikationen aus USA und Kanada zeigen einheitlich, dass stattgehabte oder aktuelle körperliche Misshandlung oder sexueller Missbrauch durch den Partner oder einen Fremden bedeutende Risikofaktoren für mütterlichen Alkoholkonsum in der Schwangerschaft darstellen.

Zwei Publikationen weisen außerdem darauf hin, dass auch emotionale Misshandlung zu Alkoholkonsum der Schwangeren führen kann.

In der Literatur finden sich viele Publikationen, die als Risikofaktoren für mütterlichen Alkoholkonsum übereinstimmend psychische oder psychiatrische Störungen gefunden haben. Zu diesen Störungen gehören vor allem die Depression, aber auch Angststörungen, Panikstörungen und sexuelle Funktionsstörungen.

Lediglich aus der amerikanischen Literatur ließ sich ein Unterschied zwischen Risikofaktoren für jeglichen Alkoholkonsum und binge drinking (exzessiver Alkoholkonsum zu einer Gelegenheit) in der Schwangerschaft bestimmen. Dabei wurde die Alkoholmenge beim binge drinking jedoch nicht einheitlich definiert. Für binge drinking in der Schwangerschaft sind in den USA eher jüngere, weiße Single-Frauen mit hohem sozioökonomischem Status gefährdet.

3.2.2 Risikofaktoren für mütterlichen Alkoholkonsum in der Schwangerschaft in Europa

Literatur: ▶ Anhang 1

Alter

Auch in Europa scheinen ältere Schwangere ein höheres Risiko für Alkoholkonsum zu haben. Häufig wird jedoch keine genaue Angabe von Lebensjahren gemacht oder eine unterschiedliche Definition von „älter" mit einem Range von > 25 Jahren bis > 30 Jahren vorgenommen.

Nationalität

Frauen ohne Migrationshintergrund haben ein höheres Risiko, Alkohol während der Schwangerschaft zu konsumieren.

Gesundheitsbezogene Risikofaktoren

Auch in den europäischen Studien werden Alkoholkonsum und binge drinking vor der Schwangerschaft als Risikofaktor für Alkoholkonsum während der Schwangerschaft bestimmt.

Frauen, die vor der Schwangerschaft Drogen oder während der Schwangerschaft Drogen oder Nikotin konsumieren, haben ein durch mehrere Publikationen übereinstimmend belegtes höheres Risiko während der Schwangerschaft Alkohol zu trinken.

Ein Artikel gibt den Hinweis darauf, dass übergewichtige Frauen eher risikobehaftet für Alkoholkonsum in der Schwangerschaft sind.

Schwangerschaftsbesonderheiten

Einige europäische Publikationen finden als Risikofaktor für Alkoholkonsum der Schwangeren eine geringe Parität.

Schwangere, die eine unbeabsichtigte Schwangerschaft austragen oder vorher einen Schwangerschaftsabbruch durchgeführt haben, haben ein höheres Risiko für Alkoholkonsum.

Sozioökonomischer Status

Die meisten europäischen Studien zeigen, dass Frauen mit mittlerem bis hohem sozioökonomischem Status häufiger Alkohol in der Schwangerschaft trinken als Frauen mit niedrigem sozioökonomischem Status. Der sozioökonomische

Status wurde erhoben als höhere Bildung, höheres Einkommen, gute Jobs, nicht arbeitslos und private Krankenversicherung.

Soziale Umgebung

Übereinstimmend mit den amerikanischen Studien ergaben auch die europäischen Publikationen, dass alleinstehende Frauen während der Schwangerschaft häufiger Alkohol konsumieren als verheiratete Frauen und Frauen, die mit einem festen Partner leben.

Eine Studie zeigt, dass auch Gefängnisinsassinnen häufig Alkohol während der Schwangerschaft konsumieren.

Psychologische Risikofaktoren

Psychische oder psychiatrische Störungen sind ein in der Literatur einheitlich bestimmter Risikofaktor für Alkoholkonsum während der Schwangerschaft.

In Europa wurde meist keine klare Trennung zwischen Risikofaktoren für Alkoholkonsum und Risikofaktoren für binge drinking gemacht. Eine dänische Studie weist darauf hin, dass Frauen, die exzessiv trinken, bevor sie wissen, dass sie schwanger sind, eher jünger und besser gebildet sowie Nulliparae sind. Frauen, die auch nach Schwangerschaftsbestätigung exzessiv trinken, stammen dagegen eher aus einer niedrigeren sozioökonomischen Schicht, seien häufiger arbeitslos und Multiparae.

3.3 Risikofaktoren für die Entwicklung eines Fetalen Alkoholsyndroms

Die Risikofaktoren für mütterlichen Alkoholkonsum in der Schwangerschaft sind abzugrenzen von den Risikofaktoren für die Entwicklung eines Fetalen Alkoholsyndroms. Bei den Risikofaktoren für die Entwicklung eines FAS werden Hinweise darauf gegeben, warum eine Frau, die während der Schwangerschaft Alkohol konsumiert, ein Kind mit Fetalem Alkoholsyndrom gebärt, während eine andere Alkohol konsumierende Schwangere ein gesundes Kind zur Welt bringt.

In diesem Teilbereich der fokussierten Literaturrecherche wurden 80 Abstracts gefunden. Davon wurden 32 Publikationen eingeschlossen (▶ **Anhang 1**).

3.3.1 Risikofaktoren für die Entwicklung eines Fetalen Alkoholsyndroms

Literatur: ▶ Anhang 1

Höhe des Alkoholkonsums

Hoher Alkoholkonsum ist laut Literaturlage assoziiert mit reduziertem Wachstum (Kopfumfang, Gehirn, Femurlänge), reduzierten sozialen und kognitiven Kompetenzen (Anzahl der Getränke pro Anlass als sensitivster Faktor für Gedächtnis- und Aufmerksamkeitsdefizite), veränderten Wachstumshormonspiegeln und Neurotransmittern.

Signifikanter Alkoholkonsum wurde in den Publikationen allerdings unterschiedlich definiert: 48 g Ethanol/d, 140 g Ethanol/Woche, 4–5 Getränke/Anlass mind. 1x/Woche oder 14 Getränke/Woche, 5 Getränke/Tag, 4–6 Getränke/Woche, > 0.5 oz Ethanol/Tag, 10 Getränke/Woche oder 45 Getränke/Monat (1 Drink=12 g Alkohol), > 3 Getränke/Woche, 140 ml Alkohol/Woche oder 630 ml/Monat.

Chronischer Alkoholkonsum ist mit einem höheren Risiko, ein Kind mit FAS zu gebären, assoziiert.

Zeitpunkt des Alkoholkonsums

Frauen, die im ersten und zweiten Trimenon Alkohol trinken, haben ein höheres Risiko ein Kind mit FAS zu gebären als solche, die nur im dritten Trimenon trinken. Bei Frauen, die nur im ersten Trimenon trinken, sind die Daten über die Gefahr der Alkoholschädigung des Kindes uneinheitlich, auch wenn häufig darauf hingewiesen wird, dass die Vulnerabilität des embryofetalen Gehirns im ersten Trimenon am höchsten ist.

Wichtig ist, dass ein höheres Risiko für FAS bei Alkoholkonsum in der gesamten Schwangerschaft im Verhältnis zu Alkoholkonsum nur in den ersten beiden Trimestern besteht.

Der schädigende Effekt von Alkohol auf das Ungeborene wird potenziert durch Amphetamine oder multiplen Drogenabusus.

Mütterliche Risikofaktoren

Alkoholkonsumierende Frauen über 30 Jahre haben ein größeres Risiko, Kinder mit FAS zu bekommen als jüngere Frauen. Die Ursachen dafür sind unklar. Hypothesen sind, dass dabei eine verminderte Alkohol-Abbaukapazität der Leber, ein insgesamt längerer und häufigerer Alkoholkonsum aufgrund des Lebensalters und eine insgesamt wahrscheinlichere Gesundheitsgefährdung älterer Schwangerer eine Rolle spielen.

Afro-Amerikaner und amerikanische Ureinwohner (Native Indians) haben ein größeres Risiko bei Alkoholkonsum ein Kind mit FAS zu gebären. Dies könnte an der unterschiedlichen Enzymkapazität der verschiedenen Ethnizitäten liegen oder aber an anderen Risikofaktoren, die in diesen Populationen häufiger vorkommen wie Unterernährung und geringer sozioökonomischer Status.

Mütter mit geringem sozioökonomischen Status, Unterernährung oder Mangel an Zink oder Folsäure haben ein höheres Risiko bei Alkoholkonsum in der Schwangerschaft ihr Kind nachhaltig zu schädigen.

Auch Stress der Mutter scheint ein Risikofaktor für die Entwicklung eines FAS beim Kind zu sein.

Alkoholinduzierte Veränderungen endokrinologischer Funktionen bei der Mutter und vorherige Geburt eines Kindes mit FAS sind Hinweise auf exzessiven oder langfristigen Alkoholkonsum der Mutter und prädestinieren für die Geburt eines weiteren Kindes mit FAS.

Geburtshilfliche Komplikationen werden ebenfalls als Risikofaktoren für die Entwicklung eines FAS angesehen. Dabei ist wahrscheinlich davon auszugehen, dass die alkoholbedingte Gehirnschädigung durch Geburtskomplikationen potenziert und somit das Outcome des Kindes insgesamt schlechter wird.

In letzter Zeit wurden viele Studien durchgeführt, die eine genetische Veranlagung für die Entstehung von FAS beforschen. Grund dafür ist, dass das FAS häufig über Generationen hinweg auftritt, dabei aber nicht immer gleich ausgeprägt sein muss (genaue Angaben über die Menge des Alkoholkonsums liegen aber häufig nicht vor). In anderen Familien, in denen höhere Mengen Alkohol auch während der Schwangerschaft konsumiert werden, tritt dagegen kein FAS auf. Bisher konnten als eventuell bedeutend für die Vulnerabilität hinsichtlich des FAS Gen-Polymorphismen für die Alkoholdehydrogenase-Enzyme ADH1B gefunden werden. Dabei scheinen ADH1B2 und ADH1B3 eine protektive Funktion auszuüben.

4 Kiterien für die Diagnose Fetales Alkoholsyndrom bei Kindern und Jugendlichen: Ergebnisse der systematischen Literaturrecherche

In den Konsensuskonferenzen wurden die Outcome-Kriterien, vor allem die Konzeptualisierung der Betreuungsaufgabe durch die richtige Diagnose zum frühestmöglichen Zeitpunkt, die Vermeidung von Fehlbehandlung, die Reduktion von Sekundärerkrankungen und die Entlastung der Eltern mehrfach bei der Festlegung sinnvoller Cut-off-Werte für diagnostische Kriterien des FAS diskutiert.

Durch die Implementierungsvorschläge der Leitliniengruppe kann eine konkrete Aufklärung von Müttern und Vätern realisiert sowie die deutschlandweite Aufklärung der Gesellschaft hinsichtlich der lebenslangen negativen Folgen von intrauteriner Alkoholexposition vorangetrieben werden.

Die vorliegende Leitlinie befasst sich mit der Diagnostik des Vollbildes FAS bei Kindern und Jugendlichen. Eine Leitlinien-Erstellung zur Diagnostik der Fetalen Alkoholspektrumstörungen ist bei noch höherer Komplexität dieser Krankheitsbilder notwendig, jedoch wegen der methodisch ungenügenden Literatur zu FASD aktuell schwer zu realisieren. Eine Leitlinie mit Empfehlungen zur Versorgung und Behandlung von Kindern und Erwachsenen mit FAS und FASD ist nach Meinung der Leitliniengruppe dringend erforderlich.

Zur übersichtlicheren Darstellung und damit besseren Anwendbarkeit in der praktischen Arbeit wurden die diagnostischen Kriterien für das Vollbild FAS bei Kindern und Jugendlichen in einem Algorithmus zusammengefasst (▶ Anhang 6).

4.1 Konsentierte Kriterien und Empfehlungen für die Diagnostik des FAS bei Kindern und Jugendlichen in Deutschland

> Zur Diagnose eines FAS sollten alle Kriterien 1. bis 4. zutreffen (Expertenkonsens, Empfehlungsgrad B, starker Konsens):
> 1. Wachstumsauffälligkeiten
> 2. Faciale Auffälligkeiten
> 3. ZNS-Auffälligkeiten
> 4. Bestätigte oder nicht bestätigte intrauterine Alkohol-Exposition.

Die Empfehlung, dass für die Diagnose FAS Auffälligkeiten in allen vier diagnostischen Säulen auftreten sollten, ist angelehnt an die bisherigen internationalen Leitlinien zur Diagnostik des FAS (▶ Kap. 2.2). Außerdem konnte in mehreren Studien gezeigt werden, dass Auffälligkeiten in nur einer diagnostischen Säule nicht ausreichend für die Diagnose FAS sind (siehe nachfolgende Beschreibung der Studien zu den vier diagnostischen Säulen).

> Bei Kontakt zum Gesundheits-/Hilfesystem sollten, wenn ein Kind Auffälligkeiten in einer der vier diagnostischen Säulen zeigt, die drei anderen diagnostischen Säulen beurteilt oder ihre Beurteilung veranlasst werden (Expertenkonsens).

Wichtig erscheint der Leitliniengruppe bei dieser Empfehlung, dass alle professionellen Helfer einschließlich Pflegepersonal, Hebammen, Geburtshelfer, Sozialpädagogen, Sozialarbeiter, Therapeuten, Diplom- und Master-Psychologen, Kinder- und Jugendlichen-Psychotherapeuten, klinisch tätige oder niedergelassene Ärzte der Gynäkologie, der Kinder- und Jugendmedizin einschließlich der Schwerpunktgebiete Neonatologie, Intensivmedizin, Neuropädiatrie, Entwicklungsneurologie und Sozialpädiatrie, der Kinder- und Jugendpsychiatrie, Psychotherapie und Psychosomatik, der Allgemeinmedizin und des öffentlichen Gesundheitsdienstes hinsichtlich der klinischen Auffälligkeiten eines FAS sensibilisiert und dazu ermutigt werden sollen, ihren Verdacht auszusprechen und die notwendige Diagnostik in die Wege zu leiten. Erst durch die Aufmerksamkeit und Kooperation aller Berufsgruppen des Helfersystems kann gewährleistet werden, dass Risikokinder einer adäquaten Diagnostik und Therapie zugeführt werden.

Die Diagnose FAS sollte bei größeren Kindern mithilfe eines Arztes und eines Psychologen gestellt werden. Bei Säuglingen und im Kleinkindalter steht die entwicklungsneurologische Beurteilung dagegen im Vordergrund. Eine multimodale und interdisziplinäre Abklärung des Kindes (wie dies beispielsweise in der Struktur eines Sozialpädiatrischen Zentrums möglich ist) ist bei Verdacht auf FAS zu empfehlen (Expertenkonsens).

Im Leitlinien-Algorithmus (▶ **Anhang 6**) wird dargestellt, dass bei einer möglichen Diagnose FAS, die jede Vertreterin/jeder Vertreter des Gesundheits- und Hilfesystems vermuten kann und sollte, das Kind zu einem FAS-erfahrenen Leistungserbringer überwiesen werden soll.

Die Leitliniengruppe verzichtet explizit darauf, diesen Leistungserbringer genauer zu definieren, da bisher keine Zertifizierung zum FAS-Spezialisten und Leitliniengruppe fordert jedoch, dass der Leistungserbringer, der die Diagnose FAS endgültig stellt, über Erfahrung mit von FAS betroffenen Kindern und Jugendlichen verfügt.

Aktuell bekannte spezialisierte Anlaufstellen für Kinder mit Verdacht auf FAS und deren Familien in Deutschland sind (folgende Aufstellung erhebt keinen Anspruch auf Vollständigkeit):

Ambulant:

- FASD-Zentrum Charité Berlin: Hr. Prof. Dr. med. Hans-Ludwig Spohr, Fr. Dipl.-Psych. Jessica Wagner, fasd-zentrum@charite.de
- Evangelischer Verein Sonnenhof: Fr. Dipl.-Psych. Gela Becker, sonnenhof-ev@t-online.de
- Universität Münster: Hr. Dr. phil. Dipl.-Psych. Reinhold Feldmann, feldrei@uni-muenster.de
- iSPZ München, Dr. von Haunersches Kinderspital, Ludwig-Maximilians-Universität München (www.spz-muenchen.com): Fr. Dr. med. Dipl.-Psych. Mirjam N. Landgraf, mirjam.landgraf@med.uni-muenchen.de
- Heckscher Klinikum München (Kinder- und Jugendpsychiatrie, Psychosomatik und Psychotherapie): Hr. Dr. med. Martin Sobanski, martin.sobanski@heckscher-klinik.de, Fr. Dipl.-Psych. Penelope Thomas, penelope.thomas@heckscher-klinik.de
- SPZ, Elisabeth Krankenhaus Essen: Dr. med. Antje Erencin, spz@contilia.de
- LVR Klinikum Essen (Kinder- und Jugendpsychiatrie, Psychotherapie und Psychosomatik), Universität Duisburg-Essen (http://www.rk-essen.lvr.de/behandlungsangebote/ambulanzen/fas.htm): Nora.Doerrie@lvr.de, Dipl.-Psych. Inga Freunscht, Inga.Freunscht@lvr.de.

Stationär:

KMG Rehabilitationszentrum Sülzhayn: Fr. Dr. med. Heike Hoff-Emden, h.hoff-emden@kmg-kliniken.de.

Rechtlicher Beistand:

Fr. Gila Schindler, Rechtsanwältin für Kinder- und Jugendhilferecht, schindler@msbh.de.

Für Informationen bezüglich Fachtagungen, Fortbildungen, Familien-Freizeiten und für weiterführende Informationen zum Thema FAS sowie für den Erfahrensaustausch betroffener Kinder und Familien empfiehlt die Leitliniengruppe, die Patientenvertretung FASD Deutschland e. V. zu kontaktieren (www.fasd-deutschland.de).

4.1.1 Wachstumsauffälligkeiten

> Zur Erfüllung des Kriteriums „Wachstumsauffälligkeiten" soll mindestens eine der folgenden Auffälligkeiten, adaptiert an Gestationsalter, Alter, Geschlecht, dokumentiert zu einem beliebigen Zeitpunkt, zutreffen
> (Empfehlungsgrad A, starker Konsens):
> a. Geburts- oder Körpergewicht ≤ 10. Perzentile
> b. Geburts- oder Körperlänge ≤ 10. Perzentile
> c. Body Mass Index ≤ 10. Perzentile

> Da Kinder mit FAS typischerweise Wachstumsauffälligkeiten aufzeigen (LoE 2c), das Messen der Körpermaße ein nichtinvasives Verfahren darstellt und keine Nebenwirkungen auf das Kind hat (Expertenkonsens), sollen das Körpergewicht und die Körperlänge bei Verdacht auf FAS immer erhoben werden (Empfehlungsgrad A, starker Konsens).
> Die Ergebnisse der vorangegangenen Messungen sollen berücksichtigt und Wachstumskurven angelegt werden (Expertenkonsens).
> Auffälligkeiten des Wachstums reichen als alleiniges diagnostisches Kriterium nicht für die Diagnose FAS aus (Expertenkonsens).

Wachstumsverzögerungen sind bei Kindern mit intrauteriner Alkoholexposition im Vergleich zu Kontroll-Kindern statistisch signifikant häufiger und durch Fall-Kontrollstudien als gut belegt anzusehen. Die Empfehlungen der Leitliniengruppe stützen sich vorwiegend auf die Studie von Klug et al. (2003) [40] und die Studie von Day et al. (2011) [30]. Klug et al. wiesen nach, dass Kinder mit FAS ein signifikant geringeres Geburtsgewicht und Körpergewicht sowie eine signifikant geringere Geburtslänge und Körperlänge aufweisen. Außerdem zeigte sich bei 22 % der Kinder mit FAS ein Body Mass Index < 3. Perzentile im Vergleich zu 3 % der Kinder ohne FAS. Die Studie weist einen guten Evidenzlevel von 2c auf. Die Studie von Day et al. (2011) [30] ergab, dass bei 14-jährigen Kindern nach mütterlichem Alkoholkonsum im 1. und 2. Trimenon das Körpergewicht und bei Alkoholkonsum im 1. Trimenon die Körperlänge reduziert ist (LoE 2b).

Aktuelle Perzentilenkurven der Wachstumsmaße für Kinder in Deutschland existieren z. B. von Kromeyer-Hauschild (2001), Voigt et al. (2006) und vom Robert Koch-Institut (2011).

Es sollte ausgeschlossen werden, dass die Wachstumsstörung allein durch andere Ursachen wie familiärer Kleinwuchs oder konstitutionelle Entwicklungsverzögerung, pränatale Mangelzustände, Skelettdysplasien, hormonelle Störungen, genetische Syndrome, chronische Erkrankungen, Malabsorption, Mangelernährung oder Vernachlässigung erklärt werden kann (Expertenkonsens).

Die Abklärung anderer Ursachen einer Wachstumsstörung (▶ Kap. 4.2) soll klinisch erfolgen. Erst bei klinischem Verdacht auf eine andere Ursache sollten weiterführende diagnostische Schritte wie die Bestimmung von Laborparametern oder die Durchführung bildgebender Verfahren vorgenommen werden (Expertenkonsens).

4.1.2 Faciale Auffälligkeiten

> *Zur Erfüllung des Kriteriums „Faciale Auffälligkeiten" sollen alle drei facialen Anomalien vorhanden sein (Empfehlungsgrad A, starker Konsens):*
> a. Kurze Lidspalten (≤ 3. Perzentile)
> b. Verstrichenes Philtrum (Rang 4 oder 5 auf dem Lip-Philtrum-Guide
> c. Schmale Oberlippe (Rang 4 oder 5 auf dem Lip-Philtrum-Guide).

> Da das gemeinsame Auftreten der drei facialen Auffälligkeiten kurze Lidspalten, schmale Oberlippe und verstrichenes Philtrum typisch für das FAS ist (LoE 1 b-), diese Auffälligkeiten anhand der Perzentilenkurven für Lidspalten sowie des Lip-Philtrum-Guide objektiv meßbar sind (LoE 1 b–2 b) und das Messen der facialen Merkmale ein nichtinvasives Verfahren darstellt und somit keine Nebenwirkungen für das Kind hat (Expertenkonsens), sollen die Lidspaltenlänge, das Philtrum und die Oberlippe bei Verdacht auf FAS mithilfe der Perzentilenkurven und des Lip-Philtrum-Guide beurteilt werden (Empfehlungsgrad A, starker Konsens).

Bereits Jones et al. (1976) [39] konstatierten, dass Kinder mit intrauteriner Alkoholexposition auffällige Merkmale des Gesichts zeigen. Dies wurde durch Clarren et al. durch eine Fall-Kontroll-Studie (LoE 4) 1987 bestätigt [24]. Die Festlegung einer für FAS spezifischen Kombination facialer Merkmale gelang Astley und Clarren 1995 (LoE 1 b-) [4]. Ihre Studie ergab, dass unabhängig von Rasse und Geschlecht die am besten diskriminierenden Merkmale für FAS das hypoplastische Mittelgesicht, das verstrichene Philtrum und die dünne Oberlippe sind. Dieses faciale Screening hatte eine Sensitivität von 100 % und eine Spezifität von 89,4 %. Da sich das hypoplastische Mittelgesicht nur schwer objektiv messen lässt und es großen Einflüssen durch die Ethnizität der Kinder unterliegt, wurden stattdessen die kurzen Lidspalten als faciale Auffälligkeit gewählt. Dadurch ergaben sich für das Screening auf FAS mittels der Kombination der drei facialen Auffälligkeiten verstrichenes Philtrum, schmale Oberlippe und kurze Lidspalten eine sehr gute Sensitivität von 100 % und eine Spezifität von 87,2 %. In zwei Studien gewichteten Astley und Clarren 1995 [4] und 2002 [7] die drei facialen Parameter für FAS und errechneten daraus einen D-Score, erreichten dadurch jedoch keine besseren Validitätskriterien des Screenings. Auch das Screening von Gesichtsmerkmalen mittels 3D-Laserscanner (Moore et al. 2007 [45], Fang et al. 2008 [33]), bewirkte keine größere diagnostische Sicherheit für Kinder mit FAS.

Für die Messung der Oberlippe und des Philtrums entwickelten Astley und Clarren einen photographischen Lip-Philtrum-Guide (jeweils für die kaukasische und afrikanische Ethnizität) mit fünf Fotos, die einer fünfstufigen Likert-Skala entsprechen. Anhand des Lip-Philtrum-Guide können sowohl Oberlippe als auch Philtrum des Kindes beurteilt und quantitativ eingeordnet werden (▶ Abb. 4.1). Dabei gelten Messungen mit vier und mit fünf von fünf Punkten auf der Skala als pathologisch hinsichtlich des Philtrums und der Oberlippe.

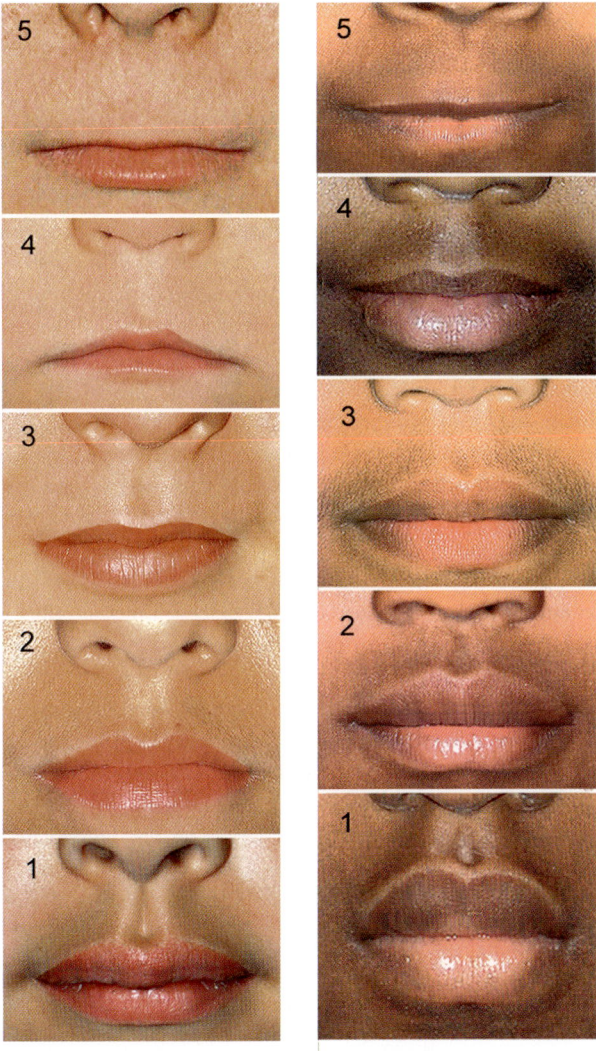

Abb. 4.1: Lip-Philtrum-Guide (© 2013 Susan Astley PhD, University of Washington)

Die Lidspaltenlänge kann mittels eines durchsichtigen Lineals direkt am Patienten oder auf einer Fotographie des Patienten mit Referenzmaßstab, z. B. 1 cm großer, auf die Stirn geklebter Punkt, gemessen werden (▶ Abb. 4.2).

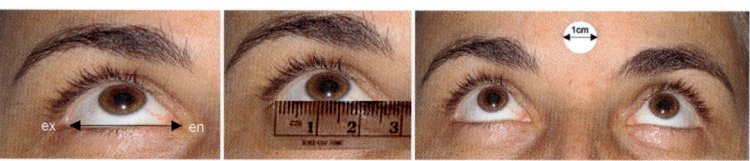

Abb. 4.2: Messung der Lidspaltenlänge (© Dr. med. Dipl.-Psych. Mirjam N. Landgraf, Ludwig-Maximilians-Universität München)

Die gemessenen Werte können in eine Perzentilenkurve für die Lidspaltenlänge eingetragen werden. Es existieren eine Perzentilenkurve der Lidspaltenlänge von Thomas et al. (1987) für Kinder von 0 Jahren (auch bereits Frühgeborene ab 29 Schwangerschaftswochen) bis zum Alter von 14 Jahren und eine Normwertkurve mit Einzeichnung von einer und zwei Standardabweichungen von Hall et al. (1989) für Kinder von 0–16 Jahren. Außerdem existieren Perzentilen von Strömland et al. (1999) [60]. Clarren et al. entwickelten 2010 [25] anhand einer kanadischen Normalpopulation (n = 2097) eine aktuelle Lidspaltenlängen-Perzentilenkurve jeweils für Mädchen und Jungen von 6–16 Jahren (LoE 2 b). Astley et al. führten 2011 eine Validierungsstudie für die kanadischen Lidspalten-Perzentilenkurven in den USA durch [12] und kamen zu dem Ergebnis, dass die Lidspalten amerikanischer gesunder Kinder kaukasischer und asiatischer Ethnizität (n = 90) im Perzentilen-Durchschnitt und die Lidspaltenlänge amerikanischer Kinder mit FAS (n = 22) mindestens zwei Standardabweichungen unter dem kanadischen Durchschnittswert liegen (LoE 2 b-). Die kanadischen Perzentilenkurven für die Lidspaltenlänge sind demnach auch auf amerikanische Kinder übertragbar. Kinder afrikanischer Ethnizität können anhand der kanadischen Lidspaltenlängen-Perzentilen jedoch nicht beurteilt werden, da der Normwert der Lidspaltenlänge circa eine Standardabweichung größer ist als bei Kindern kaukasischer und asiatischer Ethnizität. Die Perzentilenkurve von Hall et al. (1989) gibt laut der Studie von Astley et al. (2011) [12] als Normwerte zu lange Lidspalten für die jetzige Normalpopulation an.

Die Leitliniengruppe empfiehlt, zur Beurteilung der Lidspaltenlänge bei Kindern mit Verdacht auf FAS ab dem Alter von 6 Jahren die aktuellen Lidspalten-Perzentilenkurven von Clarren zu verwenden (▶ Abb. 4.3 und 4.4) (Expertenkonsens).

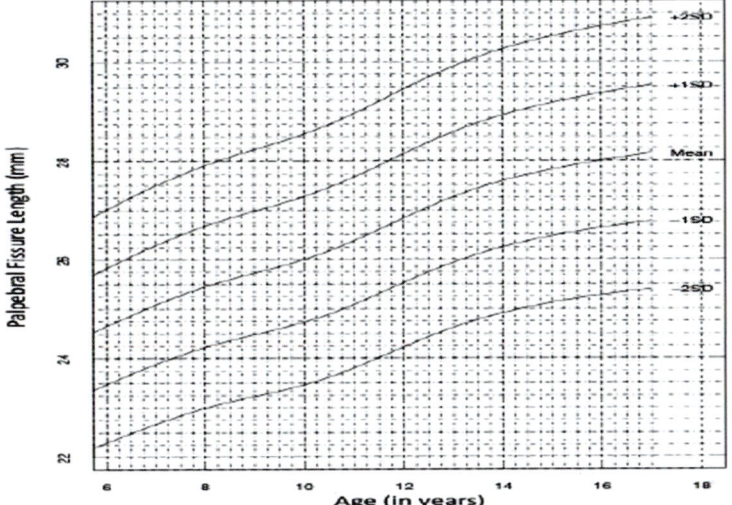

Abb. 4.3: Perzentilenkurven der Lispaltenlänge für Mädchen von 6–16 Jahren (© Sterling K. Clarren, University of British Columbia)

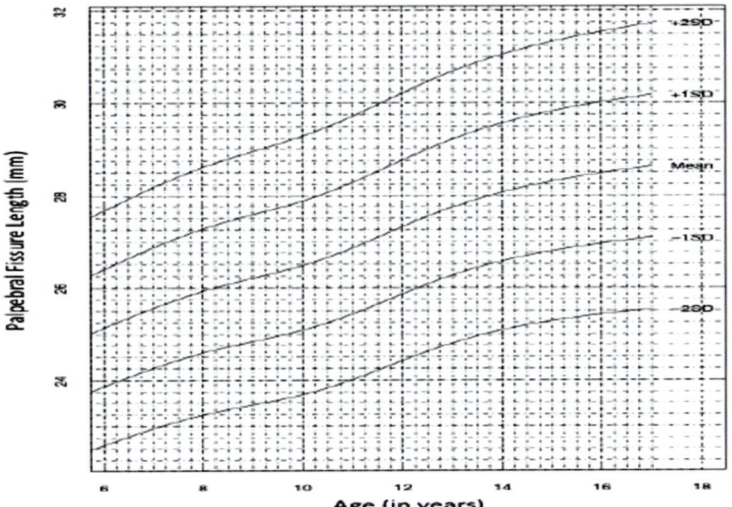

Abb. 4.4: Perzentilenkurven der Lispaltenlänge für Jungen von 6–16 Jahren (© Sterling K. Clarren, University of British Columbia)

Die Entwicklung einer aktuellen Lidspaltenlängen-Perzentilenkurve für Kinder im Alter von 0–6 Jahren hält die Leitliniengruppe für dringend notwendig.

Aktuell können für Kinder < 6 Jahre die Lidspaltenperzentilen von Strömland et al. (1999) [60] verwendet werden.

Die FAS-typischen facialen Auffälligkeiten werden bei vielen betroffenen Jugendlichen und jungen Erwachsenen mit dem Älterwerden weniger prominent und weniger eindeutig. Daher sollten bei der Diagnostik eines FAS im späteren Jugendalter auch Fotos vom Kleinkind- und Kindesalter des Jugendlichen beurteilt werden. Das diagnostische Kriterium „Faciale Auffälligkeiten" für die Diagnose FAS ist auch erfüllt, wenn der Jugendliche nur in jüngerem Alter die drei facialen Auffälligkeiten kurze Lidspalten ≤ 3. Perzentile, schmale Oberlippe und verstrichenes Philtrum (jeweils Rang 4 oder 5 des Lip Philtrum Guide) aufgewiesen hat.

> Auffälligkeiten des Gesichts reichen als alleiniges diagnostisches Kriterium nicht für die Diagnose FAS aus. Daher soll die Diagnose FAS nicht alleine anhand der facialen Auffälligkeiten gestellt werden (Expertenkonsens).

Die facialen Auffälligkeiten präsentieren die einzige diagnostische Säule des FAS, die als Screeningverfahren getestet und validiert wurde (Astley et al. 2002 [7], LoE 1 b-). Allerdings muss dabei berücksichtigt werden, dass die Evaluation der facialen Auffälligkeiten an Kindern mit FAS durchgeführt wurde, die ihre Diagnose unter anderem gerade wegen dieser facialen Auffälligkeiten bekommen hatten. Das bedeutet, dass bei den Studien kein unabhängiger Referenzstandard herangezogen werden konnte, da die facialen Kriterien bereits Teil der Diagnose FAS waren. Die Diagnose FAS soll daher nicht alleine anhand der facialen Auffälligkeiten gestellt werden.

4.1.3 ZNS-Auffälligkeiten

Zur Erfüllung des Kriteriums „ZNS-Auffälligkeiten" sollte mindestens eine der folgenden Auffälligkeiten zutreffen (Empfehlungsgrad B, Konsens):
1. Funktionelle ZNS-Auffälligkeiten
2. Strukturelle ZNS-Auffälligkeiten

Auffälligkeiten des ZNS reichen als alleiniges diagnostisches Kriterium nicht für die Diagnose FAS aus (Expertenkonsens).

Funktionelle ZNS-Auffälligkeiten

Zur Erfüllung des Kriteriums „Funktionelle ZNS-Auffälligkeiten" sollte mindestens eine der folgenden Auffälligkeiten zutreffen, die nicht adäquat für das Alter ist und nicht allein durch den familiären Hintergrund oder das soziale Umfeld erklärt werden kann (Empfehlungsgrad B, Konsens):

a. Globale Intelligenzminderung mindestens 2 Standardabweichungen unterhalb der Norm
 oder signifikante kombinierte Entwicklungsverzögerung bei Kindern unter 2 Jahren
b. Leistung mindestens 2 Standardabweichungen unterhalb der Norm entweder in mindestens 3 der folgenden Bereiche
 oder in mindestens 2 der folgenden Bereiche in Kombination mit Epilepsie:
- Sprache
- Feinmotorik
- Räumlich-visuelle Wahrnehmung oder räumlich-konstruktive Fähigkeiten
- Lern- oder Merkfähigkeit
- Exekutive Funktionen
- Rechenfertigkeiten
- Aufmerksamkeit
- Soziale Fertigkeiten oder Verhalten

Die Studien, die in den letzten 10 Jahren zu funktionellen ZNS-Auffälligkeiten bei Kindern mit FAS gefunden wurden, weisen insgesamt eine geringe methodische Qualität durch kleine Fallzahlen, fehlende Verblindung der Beurteiler, keine Anpassung bei multiplem Testen, keine Validierung am unabhängigen Kollektiv und mangelnde Berücksichtigung von Confoundern auf und erhalten somit einen niedrigen Evidenzlevel von 3b–4. Eine Einteilung der ZNS-Auffälligkeiten nach Altersklassen der Kinder ist basierend auf der jetzigen Literaturlage nicht möglich, da der Alters-Range der Studien oft mehr als 10 Jahre betrug.

Eine globale Intelligenzminderung bei Kindern mit FAS wurde in den Studien von Mattson et al. (2010) [43], Astley et al. (2009) [11], und Aragon et al. (2008) [2] gefunden.

Mattson et al. [43] bestimmten darüber hinaus zwei neuropsychologische Profile, die zwischen Kindern mit und ohne FAS besser diskriminierten als der Intelligenzquotient, allerdings mit einer relativ niedrigen Sensitivität von 78,8 % (LoE 4). Aragon et al. [2] fanden als beste neuropsychologische Diskriminatoren zwischen Kindern mit und ohne FAS die vom Lehrer bestimmte Störung der Aufmerksamkeit und die Hyperaktivität (Sensitivität 75 %). Allerdings wurde der IQ als Confounder nicht berücksichtigt, nicht zwischen FAS und FASD unterschieden und es wurden nur 4 Kinder mit dem Vollbild FAS in die Studie eingeschlossen (LoE 4). Die Studie von Astley et al. (2009) [11] ergab statistisch signifikante Unterschiede hinsichtlich funktioneller ZNS-Auffälligkeiten bei Kindern mit FAS und gesunden Kindern, aber kein spezifisches Profil bei Kindern mit FAS.

Zusammenfassend kann aufgrund der methodischen Mängel und der fehlenden Validierungsstudien anhand der jetzigen Studienlage kein einheitliches neuropsychologisches Profil von Kindern mit FAS bestimmt werden und die funktionellen ZNS-Auffälligkeiten reichen somit auch nicht als alleiniges Kriterium zur Diagnose des FAS aus.

Studien zu Leistungen in neuropsychologischen Teilbereichen von Kindern mit FAS beinhalteten entweder ganze Testbatterien oder beschäftigten sich mit nur einem bestimmten Teilbereich.

In den Studien der letzten 10 Jahre wurden in folgenden Teilbereichen Beeinträchtigungen bei Kindern mit FAS gefunden:

- Expressive Sprache, rezeptive Sprache, sprachliches Arbeitsgedächtnis oder sprachliches Lernen (Thorne et al. 2008 [61], LoE 4; Aragon et al. 2008 [2], LoE 4; Astley et al. 2009 [11], LoE 4; Vaurio et al. 2011 [62], LoE 4)
- Feinmotorik (Mattson et al. 2010 [43], LoE 4)
- Räumlich-visuelle Informationsverarbeitung, räumliches Denken, räumliches Lernen oder räumliches Gedächtnis (Mattson et al. 2010 [43], LoE 4; Pei et al. 2011 [55], LoE 4; Rasmussen et al. 2010 und 2011 [56, 57], LoE 4)
- Exekutive Funktionen (Mattson et al. 2010 [43], LoE 4; Astley et al. 2009 [11], LoE 4),

- Mathematik (Aragon et al. 2008 [2], LoE 4; Astley et al. 2009 [11], LoE 4; Vaurio et al. 2011 [62], LoE 4),
- Aufmerksamkeit vor allem Enkodieren und Wechsel von Aufmerksamkeit (Coles 2002 [27], LoE 3 b; Aragon et al. 2008 [2], LoE 4; Astley et al. 2009 [11], LoE 4, Mattson et al. 2010 [43], LoE 4; Nash et al. 2011 [47], LoE 2 b-),
- Anpassungsfähigkeit, soziale Fertigkeiten oder soziale Kommunikation (Astley et al. 2009 [11], LoE 4),
- Verhalten (Astley et al. 2009 [11], LoE 4; Vaurio et al. 2011 [62], LoE 4; Nash et al. 2006 und 2011 [47], LoE 2 b-; Fagerlund et al. 2011 [32], LoE 4)

Bemerkenswert ist, dass Nash et al. (2011) [47] eine Diskrimination von Kindern mit FASD (nur 4 Kinder mit Vollbild FAS) und gesunden Kindern mithilfe der Child Behaviour Checklist (CBCL) mit einer hohen Sensitivität von 98 %, aber nur einer geringen Spezifität von 42 % erzielten. Die Diskrimination mittels CBCL zwischen Kindern mit FASD und ADHD gelang mit einer Sensitivität von 81 % und einer Spezifität von 72 %, die Unterscheidung zwischen Kindern mit FASD und Störung des Sozialverhaltens mit oppositionell-aufsässigem Verhalten mit einer Sensitivität von 89 % und einer ebenfalls geringen Spezifität von 52 %. Auch wenn die Validitätskriterien nicht optimal sind, erscheint es sinnvoll, sowohl zur primären Verhaltenseinschätzung als auch zur Differentialdiagnose bei Kindern mit Verdacht auf FAS die CBCL zu Hilfe zu nehmen. Zur Unterscheidung von Kindern mit FAS und Kindern mit ADHD sollten zusätzlich Beurteilungen der visuell-räumlichen Fähigkeiten, der Exekutivfunktionen und der Merkfähigkeit herangezogen werden [Studien 14, 20, 58, 62].

Die von der Leitliniengruppe bestimmten Teilbereiche neuropsychologischer Funktionsstörungen basieren auf Studien mit geringer Fallzahl, so dass einzelne Zufallsergebnisse nicht ausgeschlossen werden können.

Problematisch ist darüber hinaus, dass die meisten Studien aus den USA oder Kanada stammen und die darin evaluierten psychologischen Tests in Deutschland nicht erhältlich, nicht ins Deutsche übersetzt oder nicht an deutschen Populationen normiert und validiert sind.

> Wenn faciale Auffälligkeiten und Wachstumsauffälligkeiten, jedoch keine Mikrocephalie, vorhanden sind, soll eine psychologische Diagnostik zur Diagnose FAS eingesetzt werden (Expertenkonsens).
> Funktionelle ZNS-Auffälligkeiten sollen anhand standardisierter, gut normierter psychologischer Testverfahren und einer psychologischen oder ärztlichen Verhaltenseinschätzung des Kindes für die Diagnose FAS evaluiert werden (Expertenkonsens). Bei der psychologischen Diagnostik sollen vor allem die bei Kindern mit FAS typischerweise betroffenen Bereiche beurteilt werden (Expertenkonsens).

> Welche psychologischen Testverfahren eingesetzt werden sollen, kann aufgrund der inkonsistenten Literaturlage nicht abschließend geklärt werden.

Für die Teilbereiche funktioneller ZNS-Auffälligkeiten wurden für die Formulierung diagnostischer Kriterien für das FAS in Deutschland durch Fr. Dipl.-Psych. Penelope Thomas, Fr. Dipl.-Psych. Jessica Wagner und Fr. Dr. med. Dipl.-Psych. Mirjam N. Landgraf jeweils Oberbegriffe bestimmt und geeignete psychologische Testverfahren evaluiert.

> Zu den Teilbereichen werden von der Leitliniengruppe verschiedene psychologische Testverfahren für Kinder und Jugendliche vorgeschlagen und hinsichtlich ihrer Gütekriterien beschrieben (▶ **Anhang 7**).

Bei Beurteilung der funktionellen ZNS-Auffälligkeiten ist zu beachten, dass viele psychologische Testverfahren erst ab einem bestimmten Alter des Kindes einsetzbar sind. Daher ist bei der Diagnostik eines FAS eine globale Entwicklungsverzögerung bis zum Alter von 2 Jahren gleichzusetzen mit einer Intelligenzminderung ab dem Alter von 2 Jahren. Das Kriterium „Funktionelle ZNS-Auffälligkeiten" für die Diagnose FAS ist demnach erfüllt, wenn bei Kindern bis zum Alter von 2 Jahren eine globale Entwicklungsverzögerung oder wenn bei Kindern ab dem Alter von 2 Jahren eine Intelligenzminderung vorliegt. Soweit möglich sollten standardisierte Entwicklungstests (z. B. Bayley Scales of Infant Development) auch bei sehr jungen Kindern eingesetzt werden. Die Leistungsminderung in Teilbereichen lässt sich im Säuglingsalter und teils auch im Kleinkindalter nur sehr schwer oder nicht evaluieren. In dieser Altersgruppe ist man bei der Einschätzung funktioneller ZNS-Auffälligkeiten und damit bei der Diagnose des FAS auf eine erfahrene entwicklungsneurologische Beurteilung angewiesen.

Der Cut-off der für die Diagnose FAS notwendigen Beeinträchtigung in mindestens drei Bereichen neuropsychologischer Funktionen wurde in einem Expertenkonsensus festgelegt. Die Begründung dafür ist, dass die intrauterine Alkoholexposition das Gehirn des Kindes global oder multifokal schädigt und sich der alkoholtoxische Effekt nicht nur auf einen abgegrenzten Bereich des Gehirns beschränkt.

Bell et al. zeigten in ihrer Studie 2010 [14], dass Kinder und Erwachsene mit FASD (n = 425) in 11,8 % eine oder mehrere Episoden von Krampfanfällen und in 5,9 % eine Epilepsie aufweisen (LoE 2c). Auch wenn in dieser Studie keine Kontrollgruppe ohne intrauterine Alkoholexposition existierte, sind diese Prävalenzen für epileptische Anfallsgeschehen deutlich höher als in der deutschen Normalpopulation. In einem weiteren Expertenkonsens wurde daher bestimmt, dass nur mindestens zwei funktionelle ZNS-Bereiche zur Diagnose eines FAS betroffen sein müssen, wenn zusätzlich eine Epilepsie beim Kind vorliegt. Bei klinischem Verdacht auf epileptische Anfälle soll ein Elektroencephalogramm (EEG), eventuell mit Provokation (nach den Vorgaben der Deutschen Gesellschaft für Klinische Neurophysiologie und funktionelle Bildgebung, DGKN, und der Deutschen Gesellschaft für Epileptologie, DGfE), durchgeführt werden.

Strukturelle ZNS-Auffälligkeiten

> Zur Erfüllung des Kriteriums „Strukturelle ZNS-Auffälligkeiten" sollte folgende Auffälligkeit,
> adaptiert an Gestationsalter, Alter, Geschlecht,
> dokumentiert zu einem beliebigen Zeitpunkt,
> zutreffen
> (Empfehlungsgrad B, starker Konsens):
>
> Mikrocephalie ($\leq$ 10. Perzentile/$\leq$ 3. Perzentile).

> Da das Messen des Kopfumfangs ein nichtinvasives Verfahren darstellt und keine Nebenwirkungen für das Kind hat, soll der Kopfumfang bei Verdacht auf FAS immer erhoben werden. Die Ergebnisse der vorangegangenen Messungen sollen berücksichtigt und Kopfumfangskurven angelegt werden (Expertenkonsens).

Day et al. 2002 [30] zeigten in ihrer Studie (n = 580), dass der Kopfumgang von Kindern, deren Mütter in der Schwangerschaft nicht aufhörten zu trinken, signifikant kleiner war als der Kopfumfang von Kindern ohne intrauterine Alkoholexposition (LoE 2 b). Die absolute Differenz nach 14 Jahren betrug 6,6 mm. Als Confounder wurden mütterliche Größe, Rasse, Geschlecht, Nikotinkonsum, Krankenhausaufenthalte und Anzahl von Geschwistern genannt. Handmaker et al. 2006 [36] fanden in ihrer Studie mittels pränataler Sonographie der Feten keinen absolut kleineren Kopfumfang, aber einen geringeren Kopfumfang bezogen auf den Abdomenumfang bei Kindern von Müttern, die nach Erkennen der Schwangerschaft weiterhin Alkohol konsumierten im Gegensatz zu Kindern von Müttern, die ab diesem Zeitpunkt alkoholabstinent waren (LoE 2 b).
Die Mikrocephalie ist nicht spezifisch für die Diagnose FAS.
Da der Kopfumfang in der kinderärztlichen Praxis jedoch routinemäßig erhoben wird, kein invasives Verfahren darstellt und keine Nebenwirkungen auf das Kind hat, soll der Kopfumfang bei Kindern mit Verdacht auf FAS immer gemessen und auf einer Perzentilenkurve für Mädchen oder Jungen aufgetragen

werden (z. B. Perzentilenkurven von Prader 1982, Voigt 2006 und vom Robert Koch-Institut 2011).

Welche Perzentile des Kopfumfangs als Cut-off für die Diagnose FAS geeignet ist, kann anhand der aktuellen Literaturlage nicht geklärt werden. Ein Teil der Leitliniengruppe äußerte die Befürchtung, dass ein Cut-off an der 10. Perzentile dazu führen könnte, dass häufiger keine neuropsychologische Diagnostik bei Verdacht auf FAS durchgeführt werden würde. Die Leitliniengruppe war sich darin einig, dass die neuropsychologische Diagnostik jedoch unabdingbar für den Alltag des betroffenen Kindes und seiner Familie ist, da sich daraus spezifische, individuelle therapeutische Konsequenzen und Unterstützungsmaßnahmen ableiten. Ein anderer Teil der Leitliniengruppe propagierte einen Cut-off an der 10. Perzentile, da sich dadurch das Bewusstsein hinsichtlich FAS schärfen lasse und aktuell in Deutschland eher das Problem bestehe, dass zu wenige Kinder mit FAS auch tatsächlich die Diagnose FAS erhalten. In den bisherigen amerikanischen und kanadischen Leitlinien (▶ Kap. 2.2). werden unterschiedliche Cut-offs für das diagnostische Kriterium der Mikrocephalie gefordert. In der letzten Konsensuskonferenz der deutschen Leitliniengruppe am 25. 05. 12 konnte über die Kopfumfangs-Perzentile, die als Cut-off für die Diagnose FAS gelten soll, kein Konsens erzielt werden.

> Es sollte ausgeschlossen werden, dass die Mikrocephalie alleine durch andere Ursachen wie eine familiäre Mikrocephalie, ein genetisches Syndrom, eine Stoffwechselerkrankung, eine pränatale Mangelversorgung, eine andere toxische Schädigung, eine Infektion, maternale Erkrankungen oder chronische Erkrankungen des Kindes bedingt ist (Expertenkonsens).

Andere Ursachen für eine Mikrocephalie sollen klinisch ausgeschlossen werden (▶ Differentialdiagnosen, Kap. 4.2). Erst bei klinischem Verdacht auf eine andere Erkrankung, die mit der Mikrocephalie in Zusammenhang stehen könnte, sollte eine weiterführende Diagnostik mittels Laboruntersuchungen oder bildgebenden Verfahren angestrebt werden (Expertenkonsens).

> Wenn faciale Auffälligkeiten, Wachstumsauffälligkeiten und Mikrocephalie vorhanden sind, ist eine bildgebende Diagnostik zur Diagnose des FAS nicht erforderlich (Expertenkonsens).
> Spezifische Auffälligkeiten, durch Bildgebung ersichtlich, sind bisher bei Kindern mit FAS nicht bekannt (Expertenkonsens).

Hinsichtlich der strukturellen ZNS-Auffälligkeiten ist problematisch, dass lediglich Fall-Kontroll-Studien mit Fallzahlen unter 100 und fehlenden Validitätskriterien gefunden wurden. Studien von Archibald et al. (2001) [3],

Sowell et al. (2001 und 2008) [59], Astley et al. (2009) [10], Bjorkqvist et al. (2010) [15] und Yang et al. (2011) [63] wurden evaluiert, weisen jedoch alle einen geringen Evidenzlevel von 4 auf.

Strukturelle ZNS-Auffälligkeiten, die bei Kindern mit FAS anhand von bildgebenden Verfahren, vor allem Magnetresonanztomographie (MRT), gefunden wurden, beinhalten eine Volumenminderung der grauen und weißen Substanz des Cerebrums und Cerebellums, des Nucleus caudatus, des Putamens, des Gyrus cinguli, des Liquors und eine Verdickung des Cortex (genauere Angaben in den Evidenztabellen im ▶ Anhang 3). Der Hippocampus war in den Studien von Archibald et al. (2001) [3] und Geuze et al. (2005) [34] im Gegensatz zur Studie von Astley et al. (2009) [10] nicht volumengemindert. Die Evidenz zu überproportionalen relativen Volumenminderungen einzelner Großhirnregionen ist nicht eindeutig.

Die beschriebenen strukturellen ZNS-Auffälligkeiten treten häufig bei Kindern mit FAS auf, sind jedoch nicht spezifisch für das Krankheitsbild FAS. Aufgrund der schlechten Evidenzlage und der fehlenden Validitätskriterien der bisherigen Studien im Bereich der strukturellen ZNS-Auffälligkeiten hat sich die Leitliniengruppe entschieden, strukturelle ZNS-Auffälligkeiten, außer der Mikrocephalie, vorerst nicht als Kriterium für die Diagnose FAS bei Kindern und Jugendlichen gelten zu lassen.

4.1.4 Bestätigte oder nicht bestätigte intrauterine Alkohol-Exposition

> Der Alkoholkonsum der leiblichen Mutter während der Schwangerschaft sollte bei der Diagnosestellung eines FAS evaluiert werden. Wenn Auffälligkeiten in den drei übrigen diagnostischen Säulen bestehen, soll die Diagnose eines Fetalen Alkoholsyndroms auch ohne Bestätigung eines mütterlichen Alkoholkonsums während der Schwangerschaft gestellt werden (Empfehlungsgrad A, Konsens).

Die Erfassung des Alkoholkonsums der Mutter während der Schwangerschaft ist besonders schwierig. Einerseits werden viele Mütter während der Schwangerschaft, häufig aus Angst vor Vertrauensverlust und Beziehungsabbruch, von den betreuenden Leistungserbringern nicht nach ihrem Alkoholkonsum gefragt, andererseits sind die Angaben der Mütter aufgrund sozialer Erwünschtheit oft unzutreffend. Da viele Kinder mit FAS in Adoptiv- und Pflegefamilien leben, ist die Anamnese über die leiblichen Eltern oft nur rudimentär. Burd et al. [19] untersuchten 2010 in ihrer retrospektiven Kohortenstudie (LoE 3 b) die Bedeutung der Bestätigung des mütterlichen Alkoholkonsums während der Schwangerschaft für die Sicherheit der Diagnose FAS. Wenn der Alkoholkonsum der Schwangeren nicht bestätigt werden konnte, zeigte sich eine höhere Sensitivität (89 % kein bestätigter versus 85 % bestätigter Alkoholkonsum) und eine niedrigere Spezifität (71,1 % versus 82,4 %) für die Diagnose FAS. Das bedeutet, dass mehr Kinder mit FAS auch tatsächlich die Diagnose FAS bekommen (richtig Positive), wenn der mütterliche Alkoholkonsum *nicht* bestätigt wird. Allerdings können bei nicht bestätigtem Alkoholkonsum der Mutter auch mehr Kinder, die kein FAS haben, die Diagnose FAS erhalten (falsch Positive). Da in Deutschland laut statistischen Erhebungen ein Großteil der Kinder mit FAS die Diagnose FAS nicht erhält und die nicht an FAS erkrankten Kinder aufgrund ihrer Wachstumsauffälligkeiten und ZNS-Auffälligkeiten einen ebenso großen und individuellen Förderbedarf haben, wird die niedrigere Spezifität bei dem diagnostischem Kriterium „nicht bestätigte intrauterine Alkoholexposition" von der Leitliniengruppe in Kauf genommen.

4.2 Differentialdiagnosen zum FAS bei Kindern und Jugendlichen

Die Differentialdiagnosen wurden in die drei Diagnostik-Säulen des FAS (1) Wachstumsstörungen, (2) faciale Auffälligkeiten und (3) ZNS-Auffälligkeiten unterteilt. Bei der diagnostischen Einschätzung ist darauf zu achten, dass in der vorliegenden Liste auf die Ähnlichkeiten anderer Erkrankungen mit dem FAS jeweils in einem dieser drei Bereiche eingegangen wird.

Die Erkrankungen in der folgenden Aufstellung, vor allem unter den funktionellen ZNS-Auffälligkeiten, können vom FAS abzugrenzende Differentialdiagnosen sein, treten aber auch häufig als Komorbiditäten des FAS auf.

Die vorliegende Liste der Differentialdiagnosen hat keinen Anspruch auf Vollständigkeit, weist aber auf häufige Differentialdiagnosen zum FAS hin.

1 Wachstumsstörungen
   1.1 Pränatale Wachstumsstörungen
      1.1.1 Fetale Pathologie (ungestörte intrauterine Versorgung)
- Endogen:
  - Fehlbildungen
  - Genetische Syndrome (z. B. Turner-Syndrom, Silver-Russell-Syndrom)
  - Stoffwechselerkrankungen
- Exogen:
  - Intrauterine Infektionen: z. B. Röteln, Cytomegalie, Toxoplasmose, Herpes simplex, HIV, EBV, Parvovirus B19
  - Strahlenexposition

      1.1.2 Gestörte intrauterine Versorgung
- Präplazentar:
  - Maternale Erkrankungen: Präeklampsie, Hypotonie, Anämie, zyanotische Vitien, Kollagenosen, chronische Nierenerkrankungen
  - Toxische Einflüsse, Nikotin, Drogen
  - Erhöhte maternale psychosoziale Belastung (Stress)
- Plazentar:
  - Plazenta praevia
  - Gestörte Plazentation (Uterusfehlbildung, Myome)
  - Auf die Plazenta beschränkte Chromosomenstörung

   1.2 Postnatale Wachstumsstörungen
- Familiärer Kleinwuchs
- Konstitutionelle Entwicklungsverzögerung
- Skelettdysplasien (z. B. Hypochondroplasie, Achondroplasie, Osteogenesis imperfecta)
- Metabolische Störungen

- Renale Erkrankungen
- Hormonelle Störungen
- Genetische Syndrome (z. B. Trisomie 21)
- Chronische Erkrankungen
- Malabsorption oder Mangelernährung (v. a. Mangel an Vit. D, Calcium, Eiweiß, generelle Unterernährung)
- Psychosozialer Kleinwuchs

2 Faciale Auffälligkeiten
2.1 Toxische Effekte in der Schwangerschaft
- Antikonvulsiva
- Toluol
- Maternale Phenylketonurie

2.2 Genetisch bedingte Erkrankungen
- Aarskog-Syndrom
- Cornelia-de-Lange-Syndrom
- Dubowitz-Syndrom
- Noonan-Syndrom
- Williams-Beuren-Syndrom (Mikrodeletion 7q11.23)
- Di-George-Syndrom (VCFS, Mikrodeletion 22q11)
- Blepharophimosis-Syndrom
- Hallermann-Streiff-Syndrom
- 3-M-Syndrom
- Smith-Lemli-Opitz-Syndrom
- SHORT-Syndrom
- Feingold-Syndrom (Trisomie 9)
- Kabuki-Syndrom
- Peters-Plus-Syndrom
- Rubinstein-Taybi-Syndrom
- Geleophysic dysplasia

3 ZNS-Auffälligkeiten
3.1 Funktionelle ZNS-Auffälligkeiten
- Kombinierte umschriebene Entwicklungsstörung
- Intelligenzminderung unterschiedlichen Grades
- Umschriebene Entwicklungsstörung des Sprechens und der Sprache
- Umschriebene Entwicklungsstörung motorischer Funktionen
- Umschriebene Entwicklungsstörung schulischer Fertigkeiten
- Einfache Aufmerksamkeits- und Aktivitätsstörung
- Hyperkinetische Störung des Sozialverhaltens
- Störung des Sozialverhaltens mit oppositionellem aufsässigem Verhalten
- Kombinierte Störung des Sozialverhaltens und der Emotionen
- Stereotypien

- Aggressivität
- Delinquenz
- Suchterkrankungen
- Reaktive Bindungsstörung des Kindesalters/Posttraumatische Belastungsstörung
- Sexuelle Verhaltensabweichung
- Schlafstörungen
- Angststörung/Panikstörung
- Affektive Störung
- Depressive Störung
- Epilepsien anderer Genese

3.2 Mikrocephalie

- Familiäre Mikrocephalie
- Genetische Syndrome (▶ 2.2)
- Pränatale Mangelversorgung, toxische Schädigung, Infektion
- Hypoxisch-ischämische Hirnschädigung
- Maternale Erkrankungen
- Postnatale Mangelernährung
- Stoffwechselstörungen
- Chronische Erkrankungen

Anhang 1:
Methodik Fokussierte Literaturrecherche Hintergrundinformationen

Die Suche umfasste den Zeitraum vom 01. Januar 2001 bis zum 12. Oktober 2011 und Dokumente in deutscher und englischer Sprache. Die fokussierte Literatursuche musste aus Kapazitätsgründen auf einige Länder begrenzt werden. Aufgrund der ähnlichen gesellschaftlichen und kulturellen Zusammensetzung wurde die Literaturrecherche auf die Länder Europas sowie die USA und Kanada beschränkt.

Die Suche wurde in folgenden Recherchequellen durchgeführt:

- Literaturdatenbank Medline über http://www.pubmed.org
- The Cochrane Library über http://www.thecochranelibrary.com.

Die gemäß den Suchkriterien gefundenen Abstracts wurden den zuständigen Mitarbeitern geschickt, die alle Abstracts sichteten. Dabei wurden anhand der vorher definierten Ausschlusskriterien weitere Artikel durch Sichtung der Abstracts ausgeschlossen oder an die Bearbeiter anderer Teilbereiche weitergeleitet. Die relevanten Publikationen wurden durchgearbeitet, zusammengefasst und deren Ergebnisse zu finalen Aussagen zusammengeführt.

Da es sich bei den Ergebnissen der fokussierten Literaturrecherche nicht um die Haupt-Fragestellung der Leitlinie (Diagnostik des FAS) sondern um Hintergrundinformationen für die Leitlinie handelt, wurde keine formale Bewertung der Studien bezüglich Studiendurchführung, Anzahl der Teilnehmer und Berücksichtigung möglicher Fehlerquellen sowie keine Evidenzbewertung der Literatur durchgeführt und es wurden keine evidenzbasierten Empfehlungen abgeleitet.

Teilbereich 1: Epidemiologie

Als Recherchevokabular wurden folgende Begriffe verwendet:

- fetal alcohol syndrome, fetal alcohol related deficit, fetal alcohol spectrum disorders, FAS, FASD, embryopathy, fetal alcohol effects
- epidemiology, incidence, frequency, prevalence, occurrence, statistics.

Ausschlusskriterien für die Relevanzsichtung
A1: andere Erkrankung
A2: Tiere/in vitro
A3: anderes Thema

A4: keine echten Studien z. B. Leserbriefe etc.
A5: anderes Land als Länder Europas, USA und Kanada.

PubMed (12. Oktober 2011)

Nr.	Suchfrage	Anzahl
#4	#1 AND #2 Limits: English, German, Publication Date from 2001	1 914
#3	#1 AND #2	3 123
#2	epidemiology OR incidence OR frequency OR prevalence OR occurrence OR statistics (Details: ("epidemiology"[Subheading] OR "epidemiology"[All Fields] OR "epidemiology"[MeSH Terms]) OR ("epidemiology"[Subheading] OR "epidemiology"[All Fields] OR "incidence"[All Fields] OR "incidence"[MeSH Terms]) OR ("epidemiology"[Subheading] OR "epidemiology"[All Fields] OR "frequency"[All Fields] OR "epidemiology"[MeSH Terms] OR "frequency"[All Fields]) OR ("epidemiology"[Subheading] OR "epidemiology"[All Fields] OR "prevalence"[All Fields] OR "prevalence"[MeSH Terms]) OR ("epidemiology"[Subheading] OR "epidemiology"[All Fields] OR "occurrence"[All Fields] OR "epidemiology"[MeSH Terms] OR "occurrence"[All Fields]) OR ("Statistics (Ber)"[Journal] OR "statistics"[All Fields]))	2 701 325
1	fetal alcohol syndrome OR fetal alcohol related deficit OR fetal alcohol spectrum disorders OR FAS OR FASD OR (alcohol AND embryopathy) OR fetal alcohol effects (Details: ("foetal alcohol syndrome"[All Fields] OR "fetal alcohol syndrome"[MeSH Terms] OR ("fetal"[All Fields] AND "alcohol"[All Fields] AND "syndrome"[All Fields]) OR "fetal alcohol syndrome"[All Fields]) OR (("fetus"[MeSH Terms] OR "fetus"[All Fields] OR "fetal"[All Fields]) AND ("ethanol"[MeSH Terms] OR "ethanol"[All Fields] OR "alcohol"[All Fields] OR "alcohols"[MeSH Terms] OR "alcohols"[All Fields]) AND related [All Fields] AND ("malnutrition"[MeSH Terms] OR "malnutrition"[All Fields] OR "deficit"[All Fields])) OR (("fetus"[MeSH Terms] OR "fetus"[All Fields] OR "fetal"[All Fields]) AND ("ethanol"[MeSH Terms] OR "ethanol"[All Fields] OR "alcohol"[All Fields] OR "alcohols"[MeSH Terms] OR "alcohols"[All Fields]) AND ("Spectrum"[Journal] OR "spectrum"[All Fields]) AND ("disease"[MeSH Terms] OR "disease"[All Fields] OR "disorders"[All Fields])) OR ("fas"[All Fields]) OR FASD[All Fields] OR (("ethanol"[MeSH Terms] OR "ethanol"[All Fields] OR "alcohol"[All Fields] OR "alcohols"[MeSH Terms] OR "alcohols"[All Fields]) AND ("fetal diseases"[MeSH Terms] OR ("fetal"[All Fields] AND "diseases"[All Fields]) OR "fetal diseases"[All Fields] OR "embryopathy"[All Fields])) OR ("fetal alcohol syndrome"[MeSH Terms] OR ("fetal"[All Fields] AND "alcohol"[All Fields] AND "syndrome"[All Fields]) OR "fetal alcohol syndrome"[All Fields]) OR ("fetal"[All Fields] AND "alcohol"[All Fields] AND "effects"[All Fields]) OR "fetal alcohol effects"[All Fields]))	27 344

Anzahl der Treffer: 1914
Davon relevant: 450

Die Recherche ergab für die erste Fragestellung zur Prävalenz von mütterlichem Alkoholkonsum in der Schwangerschaft und von FAS in den entsprechenden Ländern 450 als potentiell relevant eingestufte Abstracts, die entsprechend der formulierten Ausschlusskriterien durchgesehen wurden.

Nach dem Screening der Abstracts verblieben 50 Studien; weitere 10 Studien wurden über die separate Recherche zum Teilbereich Risikofaktoren für mütterlichen Alkoholkonsum identifiziert. Nach dem Screening des Volltextes dieser 60 Studien wurden 27 Primärstudien eingeschlossen.

Aus diesen Studien wurden folgende Informationen extrahiert:

- Autoren
- Journal
- Land
- Population
- Dauer der Studie
- Anzahl der Teilnehmer
- FAS-Prävalenz oder -Inzidenz und Konfidenzintervalle
- Definition von binge drinking (Sturz-Trinken, Komasaufen)
- Prävalenz von mütterlichem Alkoholkonsum während der Schwangerschaft (Konfidenzintervalle wurden in den eingeschlossenen Studien nicht berichtet)
- Notizen (z. B. genauere Beschreibung der Studie, Abkürzungen)

Eingeschlossene Literatur zu Prävalenz von mütterlichem Alkoholkonsum während der Schwangerschaft und FAS

Aliyu et al. (2009) Prenatal alcohol consumption and fetal growth restriction: potentiation effect by concomitant smoking. Nicotine Tob Res 11:36–43.

Alvik et al. (2006) Alcohol use before and during pregnancy: a population-based study. Acta Obstet Gynecol Scand 85:1292–1298.

Astley et al. (2002) Application of the fetal alcohol syndrome facial photographic screening tool in a foster care population. J Pediatr 141:712–7.

Astley (2004) Fetal alcohol syndrome prevention in Washington State: evidence of success. Paediatr Perinat Epidemiol. 18:344–51.

Bergmann et al. (2007) Perinatal risk factors for long-term health. Results of the German Health Interview and Examination Survey for Children and Adolescents (KiGGS). Bundesgesundheitsblatt Gesundheitsforschung Gesundheitsschutz 50:670–676.

Centers for Disease Control and Prevention (2002) Fetal alcohol syndrome – Alaska, Arizona, Colorado, and New York, 1995–1997. JAMA 288:38–40.

Centres for Disease Control and Prevention (2009) Alcohol use among pregnant and nonpregnant women of childbearing age – United States, 1991–2005. MMWR Morb Mortal Wkly Rep. 58:529–32.

Chambers et al. (2005) Alcohol consumption among low-income pregnant Latinas Alcohol Clin Exp Res 29:2022–8.

de Chazeron et al. (2008) Is pregnancy the time to change alcohol consumption habits in France? Alcohol Clin Exp Res 32:868–73.

Donnelly et al. (2008) Illegal drug use, smoking and alcohol consumption in a low-risk Irish primigravid population. J Perinat Med 36:70–72.

Drews et al. (2003) Prevalence of prenatal drinking assessed at an urban public hospital and a suburban private hospital J Matern Fetal Neonatal Med 13:85–93.

Druschel et al. (2007) Issues in estimating the prevalence of fetal alcohol syndrome: examination of 2 counties in New York State. Pediatrics 119:e384–e390.

Elgen et al. (2007) Lack of recognition and complexity of foetal alcohol neuroimpairments. Acta Paediatr 96:237–41.

Ethen et al. (2009) Alcohol consumption by women before and during pregnancy. Matern Child Health J 13:274–285.

Fox et al. (2003) Estimating prevalence of fetal alcohol syndrome (FAS): effectiveness of a passive birth defects registry system. Birth Defects Res A Clin Mol Teratol 67:604–8.

Goransson et al. (2003) Fetus at risk: prevalence of alcohol consumption during pregnancy estimated with a simple screening method in Swedish antenatal clinics. Addiction 98:1513–20.

Grant et al. (2009) Alcohol use before and during pregnancy in western Washington, 1989–2004: implications for the prevention of fetal alcohol spectrum disorders. Am J Obstet Gynecol 200:278.

May et al. (2006) Epidemiology of FASD in a province in Italy: Prevalence and characteristics of children in a random sample of schools. Alcohol Clin Exp Res 30:1562–75.

May et al. (2011) Prevalence of children with severe fetal alcohol spectrum disorders in communities near Rome, Italy: new estimated rates are higher than previous estimates. Int J Environ Res Public Health 8:2331–51.

Morleo et al. (2011) Under-reporting of foetal alcohol spectrum disorders: an analysis of hospital episode statistics. BMC Pediatr 11:14.

O'Connor et al. (2003) Alcohol use in pregnant low-income women J Stud Alcohol 64:773–83.

Poitra et al. (2003) A school-based screening program for fetal alcohol syndrome Neurotoxicol Teratol 25:725–9.

Strandberg-Larsen et al. (2008) Characteristics of women who binge drink before and after they become aware of their pregnancy. Eur J Epidemiol 23:565–572.

Thanh et al. (2010) Drinking alcohol during pregnancy: evidence from Canadian Community Health Survey 2007/2008. J Popul Ther Clin Pharmacol. 17:e302–e307.

Tsai et al. (2007) Patterns and average volume of alcohol use among women of childbearing age. Matern Child Health J 11:437–45.

U. S. Government (2003) Birth defects surveillance data from selected states, 1996–2000 Birth Defects Res A Clin Mol Teratol 67:729–818.

Weiss et al. (2004) The Wisconsin Fetal Alcohol Syndrome Screening Project WMJ 103:53–60.

Teilbereich 2: Risikofaktoren für mütterlichen Alkoholkonsum während der Schwangerschaft

Als Recherchevokabular wurden folgende Begriffe verwendet:

- risk
- alcohol
- pregnancy

Ausschlusskriterien für Relevanzsichtung

A1: anderes Thema/andere Erkrankung
A2: Tiere/in vitro
A3: keine echten Studien z. B. Leserbriefe etc.
A4: anderes Land als Länder Europas, USA und Kanada
A5: Erwachsene

PubMed (19. Oktober 2011)

Nr.	Suchfrage	Anzahl
#2	#1 Limits: English, German, Publication Date from 2001	1864
#1	risk AND alcohol AND pregnancy (Details: ("risk"[MeSH Terms] OR "risk"[All Fields]) AND ("ethanol"[MeSH Terms] OR "ethanol"[All Fields] OR "alcohol"[All Fields] OR "alcohols"[MeSH Terms] OR "alcohols"[All Fields]) AND ("pregnancy"[MeSH Terms] OR "pregnancy"[All Fields]))	3796

Anzahl der Treffer: 1864
Davon relevant: 298

Cochrane (19. Oktober 2011)

Nr.	Suchfrage	Anzahl
#1	(risk AND alcohol and pregnancy):ti,ab,kw from 2001 to 2011	43

- Cochrane Database of Systematic Reviews: 9
- Database of Abstracts of Reviews of Effects: 0
- Cochrane Central Register of Controlled Trials: 31
- Cochrane Methodology Register: 1
- Health Technology Assessment Database: 1
- NHS Economic Evaluation Database: 1

Anzahl der Treffer: 43
Davon neu: 8
Davon relevant: 1

Insgesamt wurden bei der ersten Recherche mittels Recherchemaske 399 Abstracts gefunden, denen aus anderen Bereichen der fokussierten Literaturrecherche drei Abstracts folgten. Nach Sichtung der Abstracts wurden 60 Publikationen in die Volltextrecherche eingeschlossen.

In der Volltextrecherche wurden 38 Artikel aus den USA, drei Artikel aus Kanada und neun Artikel aus Europa (1 x Dänemark, 2 x Deutschland, 1 x Großbritannien, 1 x Irland, 1 x Italien, 1 x Norwegen, 2 x Schweden) gefunden, die Risikofaktoren für Alkoholkonsum in der Schwangerschaft bestimmt haben.

Eingeschlossene Literatur zu Risikofaktoren für mütterlichen Alkoholkonsum während der Schwangerschaft

Ahluwalia et al. (2004) Mental and Physical Distress and High-Risk Behaviors Among Reproductive-Age Women. Obstet Gynecol. 104:477–83.

Alvanzo und Svikis (2008) History of Physical Abuse and Periconceptional Drinking in PregnantWomen. Substance Use & Misuse 43:1098–1109.

Alvik et al. (2006) Alcohol use before and during pregnancy: a population-based study. Acta Obstetricia et Gynecologica85: 1292–1298.

Bakhireva et al. (2009) Periconceptional binge drinking and acculturation among pregnant Latinas in New Mexico. Alcohol 43:475–481.

Bergmann et al. (2007) Perinatale Einflussfaktoren auf die spätere Gesundheit – Ergebnisse des Kinder- und Jugendgesundheitssurveys (KiGGS). Bundesgesundheitsblatt – Gesundheitsforschung – Gesundheitsschutz. 50:670–676.

Bobo et al. (2007) Identifying social drinkers likely to consume alcohol during pregnancy: Findings from a prospective cohort study. Psychological Reports 101:857–870.

Chambers et al. (2005) Alcohol Consumption among Low-Income Pregnant Latinas. Alcohol Clin Exp Res. 29:2022–2028.

Cheng et al. (2011) Alcohol Consumption During Pregnancy Prevalence and Provider Assessment. Obstet Gynecol. 117:212–7.

De Santis et al. (2011) Smoking, alcohol consumption and illicit drug use in an Italian population of pregnant women. European Journal of Obstetrics & Gynecology and Reproductive Biology 159:106–110.

Elo und Culhane (2010) Variations in Health and Health Behaviors by Nativity Among Pregnant Black Women in Philadelphia. Am J Public Health 100:2185–2192.

Ethen et al. (2009) Alcohol Consumption by Women Before and During Pregnancy. National Birth Defects Prevention Study. Matern Child Health J. 13:274–285.

Floyd et al. (2002) Alcohol-Exposed Pregnancy. Characteristics Associated with Risk. Project CHOICES Research Group. Am J Prev Med. 23:166–173.

Flynn et al. (2003) Rates and Correlates of Alcohol Use Among Pregnant Women in Obstetrics Clinics. Alcohol Clin Exp Res. 27:81–87.

Flynn et al. (2007) Brief detection and co-occurrence of violence, depression and alcohol risk in prenatal care settings. Arch Womens Ment Health 10:155–161.

Flynn und Chermack (2008) Prenatal Alcohol Use: The Role of Lifetime Problems With Alcohol, Drugs, Depression, and Violence. J. Stud. Alcohol Drugs 69:500–509.

Göransson et al. (2003) Fetus at risk: prevalence of alcohol consumption during pregnancy estimated with a simple screening method in Swedish antenatal clinics. Addiction 98:1513–1520.

Harelick et al. (2011) Preconception Health of Low Socioeconomic Status Women: Assessing Knowledge and Behaviors. Women's Health Issues21:272–276.

Harrison und Sidebottom (2009) Alcohol and Drug Use Before and During Pregnancy: An Examination of Use Patterns and Predictors of Cessation. Matern Child Health J. 13:386–394.

Havens et al. (2009) Factors associated with substance use during pregnancy: Results from a national sample. Drug and Alcohol Dependence 99:89–95.

Hayes et al. (2002) Prenatal Alcohol Intake in a Rural, Caucasian Clinic. Fam Med 34:120–5.

Haynes et al. (2003) Determinants of alcohol use in pregnant women at risk for alcohol consumption. Neurotoxicology and Teratology 25:659–666.

Jones (2011) The Effects of Alcohol on Fetal Development. Birth Defects Research (Part C) 93:3–11.

Karjane et al. (2008) Alcohol Abuse Risk Factors and Psychiatric Disorders in Pregnant Women with a History of Infertility. Journal of Women's health 17.

Kiely et al. (2011) Patterns of alcohol consumption among pregnant African-American women in Washington, DC, USA. Paediatric and Perinatal Epidemiology 25:328–339.

Knight und Plugge (2005) Risk factors for adverse perinatal outcomes in imprisoned pregnant women: a systematic review. BMC Public Health5:111.

Kvigne et al. (2003) Characteristics of Mothers Who Have Children with Fetal Alcohol Syndrome or Some Characteristics of Fetal Alcohol Syndrome. J Am Board Fam Pract 16:296–303.

Leonardson und Loudenburg (2003) Risk factors for alcohol use during pregnancy in a multistate area. Neurotoxicology and Teratology 25:651–658.

Lucas et al. (2003) Alcohol use among pregnant African American women: Ecological Considerations. Health & Social Work 28.

Magnusson et al. (2007) Hazardous alcohol users during pregnancy: Psychiatric health and personality traits. Drug and Alcohol Dependence 89:275–281.

Martin et al. (2003) Substance Use Before and During Pregnancy: Links to Intimate Partner Violence. Am Drug Alcohol Abuse 29:599–617.

May und Gossage (2001) Estimating the Prevalence of Fetal Alcohol Syndrome: A Summary. Alcohol Res Health 25:159–67.

McGartland Rubio et al. (2008) Factors Associated with Alcohol Use, Depression, and Their Cooccurrence during Pregnancy. Alcohol Clin Exp Res. 32:1543–1551.

Meschke et al. (2003) Assessing the risk of fetal alcohol syndrome: understanding substance use among pregnant women. Neurotoxicology and Teratology 25:667–674.

Meschke et al. (2008) Correlates of Prenatal Alcohol Use. Matern Child Health J. 12:442–451.

Meshberg-Cohen und Svikis (2007) Panic disorder, trait anxiety, and alcohol use in pregnant und nonpregnant women. Comprehensive Psychiatry 48:504–510.

Muckle et al. (2011) Alcohol, Smoking, and Drug Use Among Inuit Women of Childbearing Age During Pregnancy and the Risk to Children. Alcohol Clin Exp Res. 35:1081–1091.

Mullally et al. (2011) Prevalence, predictors and perinatal outcomes of peri-conceptional alcohol exposure-retrospective cohort study in an urban obstetric population in Ireland. BMC Pregnancy and Childbirth. 11:27.

O'Connor und Whaley (2006) Health Care Provider Advice and Risk Factors Associated With Alcohol Consumption Following Pregnancy Recognition. J Stud Alcohol 67:22–31.

Orr et al. (2008) Unintended Pregnancy and Prenatal Behaviors Among Urban, Black Women in Baltimore, Maryland: The Baltimore Preterm Birth Study. Ann Epidemiol. 18:545–551.

Page et al. (2009) Does Religiosity Affect Health Risk Behaviors in Pregnant and Postpartum Women? Matern Child Health J. 13:621–632.

Perreira und Cortes (2006) Race/Ethnicity and Nativity Differences in Alcohol and Tobacco Use During Pregnancy. Am J Public Health96:1629–1636.

Pevalin et al. (2001) Beyond biology: the social context of prenatal behaviour and birth outcomes. Soz Praventivmed. 46:233–239.

Phares et al. (2004) Surveillance for Disparities in Maternal Health-Related Behaviors -Selected States, Pregnancy Risk Assessment Monitoring System (PRAMS), 2000–2001. MMWR Surveill Summ. 53:1–13.

Rebhan et al. (2009) Rauchen, Alkoholkonsum und koffeinhaltige Getränke vor, während und nach der Schwangerschaft – Ergebnisse aus der Studie "Stillverhalten in Bayern". Gesundheitswesen71:391–8.

Sharpe und Velasquez (2008) Risk of Alcohol-Exposed Pregnancies among Low-Income, Illicit Drug-Using Women. Journal of Women's health 17.

Stotts et al. (2003) Tobacco, alcohol and caffeine use in a low-income, pregnant population. Journal of Obstetrics and Gynaecology 23:247–251.

Strandberg-Larsen et al. (2008) Characteristics of women who binge drink before and after they become aware of their pregnancy. Eur J Epidemiol. 23:565–572.

Tenkku et al. (2009) Racial Disparities in Pregnancy-Related Drinking Reduction. Matern Child Health J. 13:604–613.

Thanh und Jonsson (2010) Drinking alcohol during pregnany: evidence from Canadian Community Health Survey 2007/2008. J Popul Ther Clin Pharmacol 17.

Tsai et al. (2007) Patterns and Average Volume of Alcohol Use Among Women of Childbearing Age. Matern Child Health J. 11:437–445.

Teilbereich 3: Risikofaktoren für die Entwicklung eines FAS)

Als Recherchevokabular wurden folgende Begriffe verwendet:

- risk
- alcohol
- pregnancy

Am 09. Dezember 2011 erfolgte eine erneute Recherche mit folgendem Vokabular, mit dem Ziel, zusätzliche Dokumente zu identifizieren:

- early pregnancy, late pregnancy
- fetal alcohol syndrome, fetal alcohol related deficit, fetal alcohol spectrum disorders, FASD, FAS, alcohol embryopathy, fetal alcohol effects.

Ausschlusskriterien für Relevanzsichtung

A1: anderes Thema/andere Erkrankung
A2: Tiere/in vitro
A3: keine echten Studien, z. B. Leserbriefe
A4: anderes Land als Länder Europas, USA und Kanada

PubMed (09. Dezember 2011)

Nr.	Suchfrage	Anzahl
#4	#3 Limits: English, German, Publication Date from 2001	303
#3	#2 NOT #1	580
#2	(late Or early) And pregnancy AND (fetal alcohol syndrome OR fetal alcohol related deficit OR fetal alcohol spectrum disorders OR FASD OR FAS OR (alcohol AND embryopathy) OR fetal alcohol effects)	785
#1	risk AND alcohol AND pregnancy (Details: ("risk"[MeSH Terms] OR "risk"[All Fields]) AND ("ethanol"[MeSH Terms] OR "ethanol"[All Fields] OR "alcohol"[All Fields] OR "alcohols"[MeSH Terms] OR "alcohols"[All Fields]) AND ("pregnancy"[MeSH Terms] OR "pregnancy"[All Fields]))	3818

Anzahl der Treffer: 303
Davon relevant: 71

Cochrane (09. Dezember 2011)

Nr.	Suchfrage	Anzahl
#4	#3 from 2001 to 2011	2
#3	#2 NOT #1	4
#2	(late pregnancy OR early pregnancy):ti,ab,kw and (fetal alcohol syndrome OR fetal alcohol related deficit OR fetal alcohol spectrum disorders OR FASD OR FAS OR (alcohol AND embryopathy) OR fetal alcohol effects):ti,ab,kw	7
#1	(risk):ti,ab,kw and (alcohol):ti,ab,kw and (pregnancy):ti,ab,kw	65

- Cochrane Database of Systematic Reviews: 0
- Database of Abstracts of Reviews of Effects: 0
- Cochrane Central Register of Controlled Trials: 2
- Cochrane Methodology Register: 0
- Health Technology Assessment Database: 0
- NHS Economic Evaluation Database: 0

Anzahl der Treffer: 2
Davon neu: 1
Davon relevant: 0

Eingeschlossene Literatur zu Risikofaktoren für die Entstehung eines FAS

Aros S, Mills JL, Iniguez G, Avila A, Conley MR, Troendle J (2011) Effects of prenatal ethanol exposure on postnatal growth and the insulin-like growth factor axis. Horm Res Paediatr 75:166–173.

Bakker R, Pluimgraaff LE, Steegers EA, Raat H, Tiemeier H, Hofman A (2010) Associations of light and moderate maternal alcohol consumption with fetal growth characteristics in different periods of pregnancy: the Generation R Study. Int J Epidemiol 39:777–789.

Burden MJ, Westerlund A, Muckle G, Dodge N, Dewailly E, Nelson CA (2011) The effects of maternal binge drinking during pregnancy on neural correlates of response inhibition and memory in childhood. Alcohol Clin Exp Res 35:69–82.

Canadian Paediatric Society (2002) Fetal alcohol syndrome. Paediatr Child Health 7:161–195. http://www.ncbi.nlm.nih.gov/pmc/articles/PMC2794810/pdf/pch07161.pdf.

Chudley AE (2008) Fetal alcohol spectrum disorder: counting the invisible – mission impossible? Arch Dis Child 93:721–722.

Clarren SK, Randels SP, Sanderson M, Fineman RM (2001) Screening for fetal alcohol syndrome in primary schools: a feasibility study. Teratology 63:3–10.

Cone-Wesson B (2005) Prenatal alcohol and cocaine exposure: influences on cognition, speech, language, and hearing. J Commun Disord 38:279–302.

Cook JD (2003) Biochemical markers of alcohol use in pregnant women. Clin Biochem 36:9–19.

Day NL, Leech SL, Richardson GA, Cornelius MD, Robles N, Larkby C (2002) Prenatal alcohol exposure predicts continued deficits in offspring size at 14 years of age. Alcohol Clin Exp Res 26:1584–1591.

Drabble LA, Poole N, Magri R, Tumwesigye NM, Li Q, Plant M (2011) Conceiving risk, divergent responses: perspectives on the construction of risk of FASD in six countries. Subst Use Misuse 46:943–958.

Gallot D, de C, I, Boussiron D, Ughetto S, Vendittelli F, Legros FJ (2007) Limits of usual biochemical alcohol markers in cord blood at term: a fetal/maternal population-based study. Clin Chem Lab Med 45:546–548.

Gmel G, Kuntsche E, Rehm J (2011) Risky single-occasion drinking: bingeing is not bingeing. Addiction 106:1037–1045.

Handmaker NS, Rayburn WF, Meng C, Bell JB, Rayburn BB, Rappaport VJ (2006) Impact of alcohol exposure after pregnancy recognition on ultrasonographic fetal growth measures. Alcohol Clin Exp Res 30:892–898.

Hellemans KG, Sliwowska JH, Verma P, Weinberg J (2010) Prenatal alcohol exposure: fetal programming and later life vulnerability to stress, depression and anxiety disorders. Neurosci Biobehav Rev 34:791–807.

Isayama RN, Leite PE, Lima JP, Uziel D, Yamasaki EN (2009) Impact of ethanol on the developing GABAergic system. Anat Rec (Hoboken) 292:1922–1939.

Jones KL (2011) The effects of alcohol on fetal development. Birth Defects Res C Embryo Today 93:3–11.

Keen CL, Uriu-Adams JY, Skalny A, Grabeklis A, Grabeklis S, Green K (2010) The plausibility of maternal nutritional status being a contributing factor to the risk for fetal alcohol spectrum disorders: the potential influence of zinc status as an example. Biofactors 36:125–135.

Khaole NC, Ramchandani VA, Viljoen DL, Li TK (2004) A pilot study of alcohol exposure and pharmacokinetics in women with or without children with fetal alcohol syndrome. Alcohol Alcohol 39:503–508.

Korkman M, Kettunen S, utti-Ramo I (2003) Neurocognitive impairment in early adolescence following prenatal alcohol exposure of varying duration. Child Neuropsychol 9:117–128.

Loock C, Conry J, Cook JL, Chudley AE, Rosales T (2005) Identifying fetal alcohol spectrum disorder in primary care. CMAJ 172:628–630.

Mancinelli R, Binetti R, Ceccanti M (2006) Female drinking, environment and biological markers. Ann Ist Super Sanita 42:31–38.

McGee CL, Bjorkquist OA, Price JM, Mattson SN, Riley EP (2009) Social information processing skills in children with histories of heavy prenatal alcohol exposure. J Abnorm Child Psychol 37:817–830.

Niccols A (2007) Fetal alcohol syndrome and the developing socio-emotional brain. Brain Cogn 65:135–142.

Poitra BA, Marion S, Dionne M, Wilkie E, Dauphinais P, Wilkie-Pepion M (2003) A school-based screening program for fetal alcohol syndrome. Neurotoxicol Teratol 25:725–729.

Riikonen RS, Nokelainen P, Valkonen K, Kolehmainen AI, Kumpulainen KI, Kononen M (2005) Deep serotonergic and dopaminergic structures in fetal alcoholic syndrome: a study with nor-beta-CIT-single-photon emission computed tomography and magnetic resonance imaging volumetry. Biol Psychiatry 57:1565–1572.

Riley EP, Mattson SN, Li TK, Jacobson SW, Coles CD, Kodituwakku PW (2003) Neurobehavioral consequences of prenatal alcohol exposure: an international perspective. Alcohol Clin Exp Res 27:362–373.

Thomas JD, Zhou FC, Kane CJ (2009) Proceedings of the 2008 annual meeting of the Fetal Alcohol Spectrum Disorders Study Group. Alcohol 43:333–339.

Van Der LM, Van DK, Kleinhout M, Phaff J, De Groot CJ, De GL (2001) Infants exposed to alcohol prenatally: outcome at 3 and 7 months of age. Ann Trop Paediatr 21:127–134.

Warren KR, Li TK (2005) Genetic polymorphisms: impact on the risk of fetal alcohol spectrum disorders. Birth Defects Res A Clin Mol Teratol 73:195–203.

Zhang X, Sliwowska JH, Weinberg J (2005) Prenatal alcohol exposure and fetal programming: effects on neuroendocrine and immune function. Exp Biol Med (Maywood) 230:376–388.

Anhang 2:
Methodik Systematische Literaturrecherche Diagnostische Kriterien

Für die Sichtung der Abstracts im Rahmen der systematischen Literaturrecherche wurden prospektiv Ein- und Ausschlusskriterien festgelegt.

Einschlusskriterien

Population	Kinder und Jugendliche (< 18 Jahre) mit FAS
Intervention	Diagnostische Tests zu den folgenden Kriterien: • Wachstumsstörungen • Faciale Auffälligkeiten • ZNS-Anomalien • Alkoholkonsum der Mutter
Kontrolle	Gesunde Kinder/Jugendliche Kinder/Jugendliche mit einer diagnostizierten anderen neuropsychologischen Störung (ADHS) Kinder/Jugendliche mit anderen Fetalen Alkoholspektrumstörungen außer dem Vollbild-FAS
Endpunkte	Haupt-Zielgröße war die Sicherheit der diagnostischen Diskriminierung der eingesetzten Testverfahren im Hinblick auf die Diagnose Fetales Alkoholsyndrom. Weitere Zielgrößen wurden nicht festgelegt
Studientypen	Einschluss von randomisierten kontrollierten Studien, nachrangig Einschluss von Kohortenstudien oder Fall-Kontrollstudien bzw. Fallserien (> 10 Patienten) bzw. systematische Reviews bzw. Metaanalysen dieser Studien Anmerkung: Bei der 2. Sichtung der Volltexte wurden Fallserien ausgeschlossen
Sprachen	Englisch, Deutsch

Ausschlusskriterien auf Abstract- und Volltextebene

A1	andere Erkrankung
A2	Studien an Tieren/in vitro
A3	anderes Thema (nicht Diagnose oder Screening des FAS)
A4	Methodik der Publikation, anderer Publikationstyp
A5	unsystematischer Review
A6	Alter der Probanden überwiegend > 18 Jahre (mehr als 80 %)
A7	zum Thema Alkoholkonsum der Mutter: Publikation vor 2008 (da systematischer Review von Elliot et al [31] mit Literaturrecherche bis Juli 2008)
A8	Doppelpublikationen (Dubletten)

Bezüglich der einzuschließenden Studientypen wurde zunächst nach randomisierten kontrollierten Studien und systematischen Übersichtsarbeiten gesucht. Da vermutet wurde, dass zum Themenkomplex Diagnostik des FAS wenig randomisierte Studien existieren, wurde die Suche im zweiten Schritt bezüglich des Einschlusskriteriums Studienmethodik erweitert.

Folgende Datenbanken wurden für die systematische Suche genutzt:

- PubMed (Internetportal der National Library of Medicine, http://www.pubmed.org)
- Datenbanken der Cochrane Library (http://www.thecochranelibrary.com)

Nach Rücksprache mit der Leitlinienkoordinatorin bezüglich der Suchstrategie wurde die erste Recherche zur Diagnostik vom 10. 10. 2011 am 31. 10. 2011 mit angepassten Suchbegriffen wiederholt.

Die Recherche umfasste den Zeitraum von 01. 01. 2001 bis 31. 10. 2011. Es gab im Verlauf der Berichterstellung ein besonderes Interesse der Leitliniengruppe an Publikationen vor dem genannten Recherchezeitraum zu facialen Kriterien. Zur Identifizierung dieser Publikationen wurde in Absprache mit der Leitlinienkoordinatorin in den Referenzen der identifizierten Publikationen sowie in Pubmed-Referenzen gesucht.

Die systematische Recherche in Pubmed ergab insgesamt 1363 Treffer. Die Suche in den Datenbanken der Cochrane Library ergab 20 Treffer. Nach Sichtung von Titel und Abstract der identifizierten Publikationen wurden insgesamt 326 Publikationen eingeschlossen und zur Volltextsichtung bestellt. Die Volltexte wurden sechs verschiedenen Themenbereichen (allgemeine Texte, Wachstumsauffälligkeiten, faciale Auffälligkeiten, strukturelle ZNS-Auffälligkeiten, funktionelle ZNS-Auffälligkeiten, Alkoholkonsum der Mutter) zugeordnet und dann nach den festgelegten Ausschlusskriterien gesichtet. Die Sichtung der Volltexte führte zum Ausschluss von 148 weiteren Publikationen, sodass insgesamt 178 Publikationen zur Evidenzbewertung eingeschlossen wurden.

Recherchestrategie in Pubmed am 31. Oktober 2011

Nr.	Suchfrage	Anzahl
#6	#1 AND #4 Limits: English, German, Publication Date from 2001	1 363
#5	#1 AND #4	3 480
#4	#2 OR #3	7 693 746
#3	(developmental AND (defect OR defects OR abnormality OR abnormalities OR anomaly OR anomalies)) OR deficits OR growth deficiency OR facial phenotype OR ("central nervous system" AND (damage OR dysfunction)) OR ((cognitive OR communication OR behavioral) AND (difficulties OR disabilities)) OR adverse life outcomes OR mental health concerns OR ((fluency OR articulation) OR abilities) (Details: (developmental[All Fields] AND (defect[All Fields] OR ("abnormalities"[Subheading] OR "abnormalities"[All Fields] OR "defects"[All Fields]) OR abnormality[All Fields] OR ("abnormali-	234 689

Nr.	Suchfrage	Anzahl
	ties"[Subheading] OR "abnormalities"[All Fields] OR "congenital abnormalities"[MeSH Terms] OR ("congenital"[All Fields] AND "abnormalities"[All Fields]) OR "congenital abnormalities"[All Fields]) OR anomaly[All Fields] OR ("abnormalities"[Subheading] OR "abnormalities"[All Fields] OR "anomalies"[All Fields]))) OR deficits [All Fields] OR (("growth and development"[Subheading] OR ("growth"[All Fields] AND "development"[All Fields]) OR "growth and development"[All Fields] OR "growth"[All Fields] OR "growth"[MeSH Terms]) AND ("deficiency"[Subheading] OR "deficiency"[All Fields])) OR (("face"[MeSH Terms] OR "face"[All Fields] OR "facial"[All Fields]) AND ("phenotype"[MeSH Terms] OR "phenotype"[All Fields])) OR ("central nervous system"[All Fields] AND (damage[All Fields] OR ("physiopathology"[Subheading] OR "physiopathology"[All Fields] OR "dysfunction"[All Fields]))) OR ((cognitive[All Fields] OR ("communication"[MeSH Terms] OR "communication"[All Fields]) OR ("behavior"[MeSH Terms] OR "behavior"[All Fields] OR "behavioral"[All Fields])) AND (difficulties[All Fields] OR disabilities[All Fields])) OR (adverse[All Fields] AND ("life"[MeSH Terms] OR "life"[All Fields]) AND outcomes[All Fields]) OR (("mental health"[MeSH Terms] OR ("mental"[All Fields] AND "health"[All Fields]) OR "mental health"[All Fields]) AND concerns[All Fields]) OR ((fluency[All Fields] OR ("joints"[MeSH Terms] OR "joints"[All Fields] OR "articulation"[All Fields])) AND ("aptitude"[MeSH Terms] OR "aptitude"[All Fields] OR "abilities"[All Fields])))	
2	diagnostic OR diagnosis OR diagnoses OR screening ("diagnosis"[MeSH Terms] OR "diagnosis"[All Fields] OR "diagnostic"[All Fields]) OR ("diagnosis"[Subheading] OR "diagnosis"[All Fields] OR "diagnosis"[MeSH Terms]) OR ("diagnosis"[MeSH Terms] OR "diagnosis"[All Fields] OR "diagnoses"[All Fields]) OR ("diagnosis"[Subheading] OR "diagnosis"[All Fields] OR "screening"[All Fields] OR "mass screening"[MeSH Terms] OR "mass"[All Fields] AND "screening"[All Fields]) OR "mass screening"[All Fields] OR "screening"[All Fields])	7 587 987
1	fetal alcohol syndrome OR fetal alcohol related deficit OR fetal alcohol spectrum disorders OR FASD OR (alcohol AND embryopathy) OR fetal alcohol effects (Details: ("foetal alcohol syndrome"[All Fields] OR "fetal alcohol syndrome"[MeSH Terms] OR ("fetal"[All Fields] AND "alcohol"[All Fields] AND "syndrome"[All Fields]) OR "fetal alcohol syndrome"[All Fields]) OR (("fetus"[MeSH Terms] OR "fetus"[All Fields] OR "fetal"[All Fields]) AND ("ethanol"[MeSH Terms] OR "ethanol"[All Fields] OR "alcohol"[All Fields] OR "alcohols"[MeSH Terms] OR "alcohols"[All Fields]) AND related[All Fields] AND ("malnutrition"[MeSH Terms] OR malnutrition"[All Fields] OR "deficit"[All Fields])) OR (("fetus"[MeSH Terms] OR "fetus"[All Fields] OR "fetal"[All Fields]) AND ("ethanol"[MeSH Terms] OR "ethanol"[All Fields] OR "alcohol"[All Fields] OR "alcohols"[MeSH Terms] OR "alcohols"[All Fields]) AND ("Spectrum"[Journal] OR "spectrum"[All Fields]) AND ("disease"[MeSH Terms] OR "disease"[All Fields] OR "disorders"[All Fields])) OR FASD[All Fields] OR (("ethanol"[MeSH Terms] OR "ethanol"[All Fields] OR "alcohol"[All Fields] OR "alcohols"[MeSH Terms] OR "alcohols"[All Fields]) AND ("fetal diseases"[MeSH Terms] OR ("fetal"[All Fields] AND "diseases"[All Fields]) OR "fetal diseases"[All Fields] OR "embryopathy"[All Fields])) OR ("fetal alcohol syndrome"[MeSH Terms] OR ("fetal"[All Fields] AND "alcohol"[All Fields] AND "syndrome"[All Fields]) OR "fetal alcohol syndrome"[All Fields] OR ("fetal"[All Fields] AND "alcohol"[All Fields] AND "effects"[All Fields]) OR "fetal alcohol effects"[All Fields] Fields])	5 953

Recherchestrategie in Cochrane Library am 31. Oktober 2011

Nr.	Suchfrage	Anzahl
#3	#1 AND #2 from 2001 to 2011	20
#2	(developmental AND (defect OR defects OR abnormality OR abnormalities OR anomaly OR anomalies)) OR deficits OR growth deficiency OR facial phenotype OR ("central nervous system" AND (damage OR dysfunction)) OR ((cognitive OR communication OR behavioral) AND (difficulties OR disabilities)) OR adverse life outcomes OR mental health concerns OR ((fluency OR articulation) AND abilities) in Title, Abstract or Keywords or diagnostic OR diagnosis OR diagnoses OR screening in Title, Abstract or Keywords	85 863
#1	fetal alcohol syndrome OR fetal alcohol related deficit OR fetal alcohol spectrum disorders OR FASD OR (alcohol AND embryopathy) OR fetal alcohol effects in Title, Abstract or Keywords	46

- Cochrane Database of Systematic Reviews: 3
- Database of Abstracts of Reviews of Effects: 1
- Cochrane Central Register of Controlled Trials: 14
- Cochrane Methodology Register: 0
- Health Technology Assessment Database: 1
- NHS Economic Evaluation Database: 1

Anzahl der Treffer insgesamt: 20

Von den Volltextpublikationen wurden im ersten Schritt alle Reviews mit Angabe einer systematischen Suchstrategie extrahiert (n = 10). Zwei dieser Reviews enthielten Angaben zu allen Kriterien des FAS [39, 46], die anderen zu Teilaspekten.

Im Weiteren wurden Einzelstudien zu den Themen Wachstumsstörungen (n = 3), faciale Auffälligkeiten (n = 5), funktionelle (n = 20) und strukturelle (n = 5) ZNS-Störungen (n = 19) sowie Gewichtung des Alkoholkonsums der Mutter (n = 1) bewertet, an denen die aktuelle Evidenzlage zu dem jeweiligen Thema verdeutlicht werden kann. Es wurden überwiegend Studien berücksichtigt, die nach dem Rechercheschlussdatum der Reviews mit Angabe systematischer Recherchestrategie publiziert wurden.

Im ersten Schritt wurden Studien mit Angabe von Testgüteparametern (z. B. Sensitivität, Spezifität) berücksichtigt (n = 1 zum Kriterium „Wachstumsauffälligkeiten", n = 4 zum Kriterium „Faciale Auffälligkeiten", n = 4 zum Kriterium „Funktionelle ZNS-Auffälligkeiten" und n = 1 zur Gewichtung des Alkoholkonsums der Mutter während der Schwangerschaft). Im zweiten Schritt wurden weitere Studien eingeschlossen, die zusätzliche Aspekte der diagnostischen Kriterien abbildeten, aber nur Korrelationen oder signifikante Unterschiede von FAS-Betroffenen im Vergleich zu Kontrollen auswiesen (n = 2 zu „Wachstumsauffälligkeiten", n = 5 zu „faciale Auffälligkeiten", n = 16 zu „Funktionelle ZNS-Auffälligkeiten", n = 5 zu „Strukturelle ZNS-Auffälligkeiten"). Zu „Funktionelle ZNS-Auffälligkeiten" wurden dabei die 2010 und 2011 publizierten Studien bewertet und extrahiert. Zu „Faciale Auffälligkeiten" wurden drei Studien berücksichtigt, die vor 2001 publiziert wurden, um den Prozess der Bestimmung und später auch Messung der für FAS typischen facialen Auffälligkeiten zu verdeutlichen. Aus Ressourcengründen konnten nicht alle identifizierten Studien berücksichtigt werden.

Anhang 3: Evidenzklassifikationssystem nach Oxford (März 2009)

Level	Therapy/ Prevention, Aetiology/ Harm	Prognosis	Diagnosis	Differential diagnosis/ symptom prevalence study	Economic and decision analyses
1a	SR (with homogeneity*) of RCTs	SR (with homogeneity*) of inception cohort studies; CDR" validated in different populations	SR (with homogeneity*) of Level 1 diagnostic studies; CDR" with 1b studies from different clinical centres	SR (with homogeneity*) of prospective cohort studies	SR (with homogeneity*) of Level 1 economic studies
1b	Individual RCT (with narrow Confidence Interval"¡)	Individual inception cohort study with > 80% follow-up; CDR" validated in a single population	Validating** cohort study with good" " " reference standards; or CDR" tested within one clinical centre	Prospective cohort study with good follow-up****	Analysis based on clinically sensible costs or alternatives; systematic review(s) of the evidence; and including multi-way sensitivity analyses
1c	All or none§	All or none case-series	Absolute SpPins and SnNouts" "	All or none case-series	Absolute better-value or worse-value analyses " " " "
2a	SR (with homogeneity*) of cohort studies	SR (with homogeneity*) of either retrospective cohort studies or untreated control groups in RCTs	SR (with homogeneity*) of Level >2 diagnostic studies	SR (with homogeneity*) of 2b and better studies	SR (with homogeneity*) of Level >2 economic studies
2b	Individual cohort study (including low quality RCT; e.g., <80% follow-up)	Retrospective cohort study or follow-up of untreated control patients in an RCT; Derivation of CDR" or validated on split-sample§§§ only	Exploratory** cohort study with good" " " reference standards; CDR" after derivation, or validated only on split-sample§§§ or databases	Retrospective cohort study, or poor follow-up	Analysis based on clinically sensible costs or alternatives; limited review (s) of the evidence, or single studies; and including multi-way sensitivity analyses

Level	Therapy/ Prevention, Aetiology/ Harm	Prognosis	Diagnosis	Differential diagnosis/ symptom prevalence study	Economic and decision analyses
2c	"Outcomes" Research; Ecological studies	"Outcomes" Research		Ecological studies	Audit or outcomes research
3a	SR (with homogeneity*) of case-control studies		SR (with homogeneity*) of 3b and better studies	SR (with homogeneity*) of 3b and better studies	SR (with homogeneity*) of 3b and better studies
3b	Individual Case-Control Study		Non-consecutive study; or without consistently applied reference standards	Non-consecutive cohort study, or very limited population	Analysis based on limited alternatives or costs, poor quality estimates of data, but including sensitivity analyses incorporating clinically sensible variations.
4	Case-series (and poor quality cohort and case-control studies§§)	Case-series (and poor quality prognostic cohort studies***)	Case-control study, poor or non-independent reference standard	Case-series or superseded reference standards	Analysis with no sensitivity analysis
5	Expert opinion without explicit critical appraisal, or based on physiology, bench research or "first principles"	Expert opinion without explicit critical appraisal, or based on physiology, bench research or "first principles"	Expert opinion without explicit critical appraisal, or based on physiology, bench research or "first principles"	Expert opinion without explicit critical appraisal, or based on physiology, bench research or "first principles"	Expert opinion without explicit critical appraisal, or based on economic theory or "first principles"

NOTES

Users can add a minus-sign "-" to denote the level of that fails to provide a conclusive answer because: EITHER a single result with a wide Confidence Interval OR a Systematic Review with troublesome heterogeneity.

Such evidence is inconclusive, and therefore can only generate Grade D recommendations.

*		By homogeneity we mean a systematic review that is free of worrisome variations (heterogeneity) in the directions and degrees of results between individual studies. Not all systematic reviews with statistically significant heterogeneity need be worrisome, and not all worrisome heterogeneity need be statistically significant. As noted above, studies displaying worrisome heterogeneity should be tagged with a "-" at the end of their designated level.
"		Clinical Decision Rule. (These are algorithms or scoring systems that lead to a prognostic estimation or a diagnostic category.)
"¡		See note above for advice on how to understand, rate and use trials or other studies with wide confidence intervals.
§		Met when all patients died before the Rx became available, but some now survive on it; or when some patients died before the Rx became available, but none now die on it.
§§		By poor quality cohort study we mean one that failed to clearly define comparison groups and/or failed to measure exposures and outcomes in the same (preferably blinded), objective way in both exposed and non-exposed individuals and/or failed to identify or appropriately control known confounders and/or failed to carry out a sufficiently long and complete follow-up of patients. By poor quality case-control study we mean one that failed to clearly define comparison groups and/or failed to measure exposures and outcomes in the same (preferably blinded), objective way in both cases and controls and/or failed to identify or appropriately control known confounders.
§§§		Split-sample validation is achieved by collecting all the information in a single tranche, then artificially dividing this into "derivation" and "validation" samples.
" "		An "Absolute SpPin" is a diagnostic finding whose Specificity is so high that a Positive result rules-in the diagnosis. An "Absolute SnNout" is a diagnostic finding whose Sensitivity is so high that a Negative result rules-out the diagnosis.
"¡"¡		Good, better, bad and worse refer to the comparisons between treatments in terms of their clinical risks and benefits.
" " "		Good reference standards are independent of the test, and applied blindly or objectively to applied to all patients. Poor reference standards are haphazardly applied, but still independent of the test. Use of a non-independent reference standard (where the 'test' is included in the 'reference', or where the 'testing' affects the 'reference') implies a level 4 study.
" " " "		Better-value treatments are clearly as good but cheaper, or better at the same or reduced cost. Worse-value treatments are as good and more expensive, or worse and the equally or more expensive.
**		Validating studies test the quality of a specific diagnostic test, based on prior evidence. An exploratory study collects information and trawls the data (e.g. using a regression analysis) to find which factors are 'significant'.
***		By poor quality prognostic cohort study we mean one in which sampling was biased in favour of patients who already had the target outcome, or the measurement of outcomes was accomplished in < 80 % of study patients, or outcomes were determined in an unblinded, non-objective way, or there was no correction for confounding factors.
****		Good follow-up in a differential diagnosis study is > 80 %, with adequate time for alternative diagnoses to emerge (for example 1–6 months acute, 1–5 years chronic)

Oxford Centre for Evidence-based Medicine Levels of Evidence (March 2009, for definitions of terms used see glossary at http://www.cebm.net/?o=1116).

Produced by Bob Phillips, Chris Ball, Dave Sackett, Doug Badenoch, Sharon Straus, Brian Haynes, Martin Dawes since November 1998. Updated by Jeremy Howick March 2009.

Anhang 4:
Evidenztabellen zur eingeschlossenen Literatur über die diagnostischen Kriterien des FAS

Erstellt von Dr. med. Monika Nothacker MPH, Ärztliches Zentrum für Qualität in der Medizin

Tab. 1: Evidenztabelle systematische Reviews und HTA-Berichte (themenübergreifend)

Studientyp/ Autoren, Jahr	Suchstrategie Ein- und usschlusskriterien,	Welche Behandlungen wurden geprüft	Charakteristik eingeschlossener Studien/Befunde in Bezug auf Diagnostik	Methodische Besonderheiten/ Bemerkungen	Evidenzgraduierung nach CEBM 2009 (University of Oxford)	Literaturbelege
FAS all aspects, focus on prevention						
Systematic review/ Elliott L. et al, 2008 [31]	Systematic search in Medline, EMBASE, Scopus and PsychInfo databases. Review databases: Cochrane Database of Systematic Reviews, Cochrane Central Register of Controlled Trials, Database of Abstracts of Reviews of Effectiveness, Health Technology Assessment database, NHS Economic Evaluation database. HTA databases. Clinical	Aim of the whole review: evaluation of the main strategies of prevention, screening, diagnosis and management of FAS. **1. Prenatal screening: Reseach questions:** Are screening tools able to identify women at increased risk of having a child with FASD? **Intervention:** 1. Any strategy that aims to reduce the incidence of FASD	**1. Prenatal screening/screening tools: Biomarkers:** The literature search identified five publications which evaluated the ability of biomarkers to detect alcohol consumption in pregnant women (see Table 42). AST, ALT, MCV, GGT, CDT Combination of all biomarkers PAUI ACOG antepartum record WBAA, Urine Analysis There is no evidence that biomarkers are appropriate either as a screening tool in a clinical setting or as a comparator.	Only facts with regard to diagnostics were extracted for the evidence report „Diagnostik des FAS": Evidence assessment with NHMRC. Studies on fatty acid ethyl esters are not completely taken into account.	**1. Prenatal screening/ screening tools:** LoE 3–4 for this part of the review **2. Post-natal screening and diagnosis:** LoE 5 (in this part of the review the authors do not report any evaluation with NHMRC. Quality/methodol-	1. Prenatal screening/ screening tools: Biomarkers: Magnusson A et al. J Stud Alcohol 2005; 66 (2):157–164. Budd KW et al., (2000). J Obstet Gynecol Neonatal Nurs. 29(2):129–136. Stoler JM et al. (1998). J Pediatr. 133 (3):346–352. Christmas JT et al.,

Anhang 4

Studientyp, Autoren, Jahr	Suchstrategie Ein- und Ausschlusskriterien	Welche Behandlungen wurden geprüft	Charakteristik eingeschlossener Studien/Befunde in Bezug auf Diagnostik	Methodische Besonderheiten/ Bemerkungen	Evidenzgraduierung nach CEBM 2009 (University of Oxford)	Literaturbelege
	Practice Guideline: National Guideline Clearing House database; Agency for Healthcare Research and Quality; US Preventative Services Task Force, Scottish Intercollegiate Guidelines Network Library + hand searching of relevant journals. **Zeit:** < 1966 until Juli 2008 **1: Prenatal screening Inclusion criteria:** English language. All levels of evidence including existing systematic reviews and clinical practice guidelines, as well as different types of original studies will be eligible for inclusion	2. Any alcohol screening tool that has been: a) designed for use in pregnant women or designed to evaluate a woman's risk of having a child with FASD or b) designed for use in the general population but has been evaluated in pregnant women or used to determine if women are at increased risk of having a child with FASD **Comparator** Any comparator **Outcomes** 1. Reduction in the incidence of FASD 2. Reduction in alcohol use during pregnancy or in women of childbearing age 3. Sensitivity and specificity of the screening tool	**Questionnaires,** which aim to identify pregnant women with alcohol problems The pregnancy specific screening tools TWEAK and T-ACE were evaluated in seven publications: the most appropriate screening tool for use in the prenatal setting is the TWEAK or T-ACE (Level III-2) All publications which compared the TWEAK and T-ACE with other screening tools reported that these two screening tools had the highest sensitivity and specificity. The standard cut-point for „risk drinking" is a score of ≥2 using either test, however a score of ≥1 or ≥3 may be appropriate in a clinic with an unusually high or low-risk population.(S. 130) **2. Post-natal screening and diagnosis** The literature search did not identify any systematic reviews of screening or diagnostic criteria. The literature search identified three articles describing FASD or	Assessment of study eligibility by one reviewer. Data extraction by two reviewers Evidence for screening tools with questionnairs limited: small number of published studies and low-level of evidence available (Level III-2). For the assessment of postnatal screening and diagnosis literature only systematic reviews and published guidelines eligible for inclusion. Post-natal screen-	ogy of the single gle papers were not described) Methodik dieser Publikationen werden ebenfalls kaum bis gar nicht beschrieben. (da für die betrachteten verschiedenen Abschnitte des Reviews unterschiedliche Einschluss-Kriterien der Studientypen angewendet wurden und sehr unterschiedliche Studien betrachtet wurden, ist eine Gesamtbewer-	(1992). Obstet Gynecol. 80(5):750–754. Larsson G et al., (1983). Am J Obstet Gynecol. 147 (6):654–657. Questionnaire: Sokol RJ et al., (1989). Am J Obstet Gynecol. 160(4):863–870. Russell M et al., (1994). Clin Exp Res. 18 (5):1156–1161. Russell M et al., (1996). Am J Public Health. 86 (10):1435–1439. Chang G et al.,. (1998). Obstet Gynecol. 91(6):892–898. Chang G et al., J Stud Alcohol 1999; 60 (3):306–309.

Studientyp/ Autoren, Jahr	Suchstrategie Ein- und Ausschlusskriterien	Welche Behandlungen wurden geprüft	Charakteristik eingeschlossener Studien/Befunde in Bezug auf Diagnostik	Methodische Besonderheiten/ Bemerkungen	Evidenzgraduierung nach CEBM 2009 (University of Oxford)	Literaturbelege
	(controlled and uncontrolled). **Exclusion**: not a clinical study, wrong intervention, wrong outcome, not in English. **Patient population** Women at high risk of having a child with FASD (to identify tertiary prevention strategies). 2. Post-natal screening and diagnosis: **Inclusion criterias**: English language. Assessment of literature was conducted as a top level review. Therefore, only systematic reviews and published guidelines were eligible for inclusion.	**2. Post-natal screening and diagnosis**: **Reseach questions**: – Are postnatal screening tools (aimed at an individual suspected of having FASD and/or their mother) effective at identifying individuals who should undergo a full diagnostic FASD evaluation? – Do diagnostic tools increase the accuracy of FASD identification? **Intervention**: Any strategy that aims to identify an individual who may have FAS or diagnose an individual who may have FAS **Comparator**: any Comparator **Outcome**: Sensitivity und specificity of FAS diagnostics	FAS postnatal diagnostic criteria: Institute of Medicine, 4-Digit Diagnostic Code and Hoyme Updated Institute of Medicine Criteria. Two guidelines addressing screening **(Canadian FASD Referral Guidelines and Centre for Disease Control FASerral Guidelines)** and three guidelines addressing Diagnostics **(Canadian Guidelines, Centre for Disease Control Guidelines and British Medical Association Guidelines)** were identified. There was very little high level evidence available for these strategies. A review by Peadon 2008 found that the 4-Digit Diagnostic code was the most commonly used diagnostic criteria worldwide. **Results**: Two **guidelines** addressing **screening**: Recommendation that screening should occur based on identification of facial features, known exposure to alcohol or learning and/	ing and diagnosis: According to the authors of the review were the studies identified in the literature search generally of limited quality (methodology and appraisal for these references not reported) This „top level" review of the postnatal screening and diagnostic literature did not identify any publications that evaluated the accuracy of the diagnostic criteria. Conclusion of the authors is that no evidence exists for any criteria	tung nicht möglich).	Chang G et al. Am J Addict 1999; 8 (2):87–93. Dawson DA et al. Alcohol Clin Exp Res 2001; 25 (9):1342–1349. 2. Post-natal screening and diagnosis: 4-Digit Diagnostic Code Astley, S. 2004. Diagnostic Guide for Fetal Alcohol Spectrum Disorders: The 4-Digit Diagnostic Code. University of Washington Publication Services. Canadian Guidelines Chudley A et al. Fetal alcohol spectrum disorder: Canadian guidelines for diagnosis. Can Med Assoc J

Anhang 4

Anhang 4

Studientyp/ Autoren, Jahr	Suchstrategie Ein- und Ausschlusskriterien	Welche Behandlungen wurden geprüft	Charakteristik eingeschlossener Studien/Befunde in Bezug auf Diagnostik	Methodische Besonderheiten/ Bemerkungen	Evidenzgraduierung nach CEBM 2009 (University of Oxford)	Literaturbelege
	Population: Individuals who may have FAS or mothers of individuals who may have FAS		or behavioural difficulties. The CDC guidelines state that the screening should provide assistance in making the referral decision, rather than be used as a definitive screening tool. **Guidelines und articles addressing Diagnostics:** The five diagnostic approaches were broadly similar, evaluating maternal prenatal alcohol exposure, characteristic facial abnormalities, growth retardation and CNS abnormalities. All publications discussed the significant problems associated with diagnosing the less severe forms of FASD (i.e. children who did not meet the definition of FAS but had significant disabilities as a result of prenatal alcohol exposure). The diagnostic criteria and guidelines are widely used internationally, however there is no consensus on which criteria are most appropriate in the clinical setting.	terion as the most appropriate.		2005; 172(Suppl): Mar05-S21. CDC – National Centre on Birth Defects and Developmental Disabilities. Fetal Alcohol Syndrome: Guidelines for Referral and Diagnosis. 2004. Centre for Disease Control. Institute of Medicine – Stratton K et al., 1996. Fetal alcohol syndrome: diagnosis, epidemiology, prevention, and treatment. Washington: Institute of Medicine and National Academy Press. Hoyme Updated Institute of Medicine – Hoyme HE et al. A practical clinical ap-

Studientyp, Autoren, Jahr	Suchstrategie Ein- und Ausschlusskriterien,	Welche Behandlungen wurden geprüft	Charakteristik eingeschlossener Studien/Befunde in Bezug auf Diagnostik	Methodische Besonderheiten/Bemerkungen	Evidenzgraduierung nach CEBM 2009 (University of Oxford)	Literaturbelege
Mukherjee RA et al., 2006 review with sys-	Search in all major electronic databases incl. Medline, Embase, Psychlit, Ovid from 1966–2006.	Overview of following points: 1) Definition and clinical criteria of FASD and its subgroups	Only data with regard to diagnostics are referred, i. e. to point 1) and 4) and a part of 5): 1) Definition and clinical criteria	Cited „systematic reviews" such as Rasmussen et al. had not systematically searched literature	2 a–5 The review comprises studies of different	1) - Chudley AE et al., Fetal alcohol spectrum disorder: Canadian proach to diagnosis of fetal alcohol spectrum disorders: Clarification of the 1996 Institute of Medicine Criteria. Paediatrics 2005; 115(39):47. BMA Board of Science. Fetal alcohol spectrum disorders: A guide for healthcare professionals. 2007. Peadon E et al., (2008). BMC Paed; 8:12–20. FASD referral guidelines (Public Health Agency of Canada, 2005).

Anmerkung: Goh et al. 2008 wird unter den jeweiligen Themen extrahiert, da sehr ausführlich.

Anhang 4

Studientyp/ Autoren, Jahr	Suchstrategie Ein- und Ausschlusskriterien,	Welche Behandlungen wurden geprüft	Charakteristik eingeschlossener Studien/Befunde in Bezug auf Diagnostik	Methodische Besonderheiten/ Bemerkungen	Evidenzgraduierung nach CEBM 2009 (University of Oxford)	Literaturbelege
tematic search [46]	Using mesh headings: Fetal alcohol syndrome, Fetal alcohol effects, Fetal alcohol spectrum disorder and Prenatal alcohol. Databases were combined to give an overall single category with no exclusions from which further searches were combined. These included knowledge of fetal alcohol syndrome, pathology, psychology and management. References cited in published articles were also reviewed. Inclusion/Exclusion: Detailed criteria are not described Patient population: Not described	2) **Knowledge levels of fetal alcohol spectrum disorders** by the general public and health professionals 3) **Pathology** 4) **Neurocognitive Deficits** and secondary disabilities 5) **Management**	1. Fetal alcohol syndrome: confirmed alcohol exposure criteria a alcohol exposure b facial pattern of short palpebral fissures < 10 percentile, thin upper lip vermillion, smooth philtrum c evidence of pre/postnatal growth retardation d evidence of neurocognitive deficits 2 Fetal alcohol syndrome: no confirmed alcohol exposure a as above but no alcohol exposure found 3 **Partial fetal alcohol syndrome:** confirmed alcohol exposure a not all of the above features are present but neurocognitive and some facial features needed 4 **Alcohol related birth defect** a confirmed maternal alcohol consumption as well as some but not all of the facial features are present, however, the behavioural features or structural abnormal- erature (in this review methodology is not described) Quality/methodology of single studies is not described There is no description of efforts to identify publication bias. How many reviewers the studies assessed is not mentioned. Heterogenity is not discussed. P values, confidence intervals or other statistical measures are not reported.		kinds of quality (guideline, reviews, expert opinions (4digitcode) and primary studies – as far as assessable	guidelines for diagnosis. Can Med Assoc J 2005;172:S1–21 - Hoyme HE et al. A practical clinical approach to the diagnosis of fetal alcohol spectrum disorder: clarification of the 1996 institute of medicine criteria. Paediatrics 2005;115:39–47 4) - Jacobson JL et al. Alcohol Res Health 2002;26:282–6 - Rasmussen C. Alcohol Clin Expl Res 2005;29: 1359–67 - Streithguth AP et al.. Sem Clin Neuropsychiatry 2000;5:177–90 5) – Russel M. Alcohol Res Health

Studientyp/ Autoren, Jahr	Suchstrategie Ein- und Ausschlusskriterien,	Welche Behandlungen wurden geprüft	Charakteristik eingeschlossener Studien/Befunde in Bezug auf Diagnostik	Methodische Besonderheiten/ Bemerkungen	Evidenzgraduierung nach CEBM 2009 (University of Oxford)	Literaturbelege
			ities are more pronounced
5 **Alcohol related neurodevelopmental disorder** a confirmed maternal alcohol consumption with the absence of growth retardation or facial features and with the neurocognitive features being prominent.
Methods of diagnosis of facial abnormalities: note all of these require careful history taking and evidence of growth retardation to make the diagnosis:
1 **Gestalt:** facial pattern recognition requires experience and clear history. Issues of accuracy and inconsistency often found
2 **D score method:** computational method for facial pattern based on careful measurements of abnormalities: requires a high degree of training and skill restricting practice to a few
3 **4-digit scoring method and facial photographic recognition software:** applies areas of history and			1994;18:55–61
- Chan D. J FAS Int 2003;1:e9

Anhang 4

Studien-typ/ Autoren, Jahr	Suchstrategie Ein- und usschlusskriterien,	Welche Behandlungen wurden geprüft	Charakteristik eingeschlossener Studien/Befunde in Bezug auf Diagnostik	Methodische Besonderheiten/ Bemerkungen	Evidenz-graduierung nach CEBM 2009 (University of Oxford)	Literaturbelege
			facial recognition to four 4-point Likert scales to establish diagnosis. Requires minimal training and can be used easily by all in clinical settings **4) Neurocognitive Deficits** • Core areas of psychological deficits (Jacobson JL et al. 2002) • Hyperactivity • Attention deficits • Sustained attention • Focused attention • Cognitive flexibility • Planning difficulties • Learning/memory problems • New memories not consolidated • Lower IQ • Arithmetic difficulties • Receptive language difficulties • Verbal processing problems • Social understanding difficulties – Common secondary difficulties seen (Streithguth AP et al.) • Psychiatric problem (95 % have some form of diagnosable mental disorder:			

Anhang 4

Studien-typ/ Autoren, Jahr	Suchstrategie Ein- und usschlusskriterien, Jahr	Welche Behandlungen wurden geprüft	Charakteristik eingeschlossener Studien/Befunde in Bezug auf Diagnostik	Methodische Besonderheiten/ Bemerkungen	Evidenz-graduierung nach CEBM 2009 (University of Oxford)	Literaturbelege
			ADHD (attention deficit hyperactivity disorder), social and communicatory impairments, personality disorder, schizophrenia, addiction and depression. • Disrupted school experience • Trouble with the law • Confinement • Inappropriate sexual behaviour (50 %) • Alcohol/drug problems Much of this can be related to their inability to control and maintain their behaviour attributable to damage caused to their executive function abilities combined with difficulties in receptive language and inability to consolidate memories because of temporal/hippocampal damage. **5) Methods of detection alcohol consumption of mothers:** Emerging methods such as the use of routine screening tools such as TWEAK, hair sampling, or meco-			

Anhang 4

Anhang 4

Studientyp/ Autoren, Jahr	Suchstrategie Ein- und usschlusskriterien,	Welche Behandlungen wurden geprüft	Charakteristik eingeschlossener Studien/Befunde in Bezug auf Diagnostik	Methodische Besonderheiten/ Bemerkungen	Evidenzgraduierung nach CEBM 2009 (University of Oxford)	Literaturbelege
			nium testing have been suggested. However, the ethical debate around their use is in its infancy thus clarification is required before they can be recommended routinely.			
Biomarker						
Systematic review, Burd L et al., 2008 [18]	Literature search was conducted in Pubmed using the terms meconium, fatty acid ethyl esters, biomarkers and prenatal alcohol exposure. + hand searching Inclusion criteria: only peer reviewed studies utilizing analysis of meconium for the presence of FAEE in humans up through the year 2007 and all languages. Exclusion: not peer reviewed or without data on hu-	Measurement of fatty acid ethyl esters (FAEE) in meconium as biomarkers for prenatal alcohol exposure (PAE). 1) laboratory techniques 2) individual FAEE or combined FAEE 3) Cut-offs 4) Sensitivity and Specificity 5) exposure assessement for prenatal alcohol use Reported alcohol exposure serves as reference (s. remark in column of special features).	10 article were found with 6 different assessment strategies and 4 different analytical techniques. 1) Multiple laboratory techniques for detection of FAEE in meconium were used (s. table 1): – Gas chromatography/Flame Ionization Detection (GC-FID) – Gas chromatograph/Mass Spectroscopy (GC-MS) – Selected ion monitoring (SIM with GC-MS) – GC-MS/MS (tandem MS) According to the authors, tandem mass Spectroscopy is one of the most selective detection techniques. 2) A variable range of individual	Beginning of time period for literature search is not indicated. Quality and study design (control groups?) of single studies are not described. Assessment of history of alcohol exposure is highly variable, most were not assessing the time period of alcohol consumption in pregnancy (most relevant 3rd	3 b – (as without reference standard and troublesome heterogeneity)	Bearer CF et al., 2003. J Pediatr 143: 463–469. Bearer CF et al, 1999. Alcohol Clin Exp Res 23: 487–492. Bearer CF et al., 2005. J Pediatr 146: 824–830. Chan D et al., 2003. Ther Drug Monit 25: 271–278. Chan D et al., 2004. Ther Drug Monit 26: 474–481. Derauf C et al., 2003. Am J of Epedimiol

88

Studien-typ/ Autoren, Jahr	Suchstrategie Ein- und Ausschlusskriterien,	Welche Behandlungen wurden geprüft	Charakteristik eingeschlossener Studien/Befunde in Bezug auf Diagnostik	Methodische Besonderheiten/ Bemerkungen	Evidenz-graduierung nach CEBM 2009 (University of Oxford)	Literaturbelege
	mans Population: data on 2221 subjects; 455 (20.5 %) met their respective study's criteria for alcohol exposure. 502 (22,6 %) FAEE levels above the study's cut-off.		FAEE (9 FAEEs) or combinations for PAE as a positive marker were used (table 2): Ethyl laureate, ethyl palmitate etc. 3) There was also variance in the methods used to determine the cutoffs (table 3) 4) Sensitivity and Specifity (table 4) also vary. Best values were found for ethyl oleate with sensitivity of 84.2 % and specifity of 83.3 %, cut-off 0032 µg/g (Bearer et al. 2003). Thus, developing a summary estimate of the accurancy of detection of PAE of combined estimates of sensitivity or specifity was not possible. 5) Strategies for exposure assessment for prenatal alcohol use were also variable (table 5): Maternal self-reporting; medical record review, clinician suspicion;	trimester when meconium is formed, only 4 studies). Thus, consumption earlier in pregnancy is not detectable by meconium assay. Limitation of the review is the troublesome heterogeneity of measurements of the single studies. Thus, outcome measures are not comparable. Due to incompleteness of data pooling of the variables were not possible. Except for data to sensitivity and		158: 705–709. Klein J et al., 1999. Ther Drug Monit 21: 644–646. Moore C et al., 2003. Clin Chem 49:133–136 Moore C et al., 2001. Clin Chem Acta 312:235–238. Ostrea EM et al., 2006. Alcohol Clin Exp Res 30: 1152–1159

Anhang 4

Anhang 4

Studientyp/ Autoren, Jahr	Suchstrategie Ein- und Ausschlusskriterien	Welche Behandlungen wurden geprüft	Charakteristik eingeschlossener Studien/Befunde in Bezug auf Diagnostik	Methodische Besonderheiten/ Bemerkungen	Evidenzgraduierung nach CEBM 2009 (University of Oxford)	Literaturbelege
			screening questionnaire or interview, timeline follow-back approach.	specifity other statistical measures were not reported.		
			9 articles found a correlation between FAEE levels and maternal alcohol consumption, one article found not (Derauf et al.).	There is no description of efforts to identify publication bias.		
Goh I. Y. et al. 2008 Systematic Review Here extracted: underlying evidence report of the sited publication given in a link Biomarker	Search Methods: Search in Medline and Pubmed 1966 up to 12/2007 No language restriction Search terms: screening, fetal alcohol spectrum disorder, fetal alcohol syndrome Inclusion criteria: methodologies of screening for FASD in children up to 18 years, Studies of adults excluded	Different Screening methods for FAS Evaluation of Test accuracy: Sensitivity Specificity Positive predictive Value Negative predictive Value	**Biomarker** **1. Meconium** Fatty acid ethyl esters (FAEE) – true correlate, only 2.+3. trimester Quantified as linoleic, oleic, steric, palmitoleic esters. 1. Study in Hawaii prevalence 16,7 % positive 2. Study anonymous population study: 2,5 % positive 3. Study in Montevideo 44 % positive 4. Study anonymous population: 26 % positive The disadvantage of meconium screening is that there is a limited window to collect meconium. Meconium is only able to detect pre-	No description of the underlying study quality	LOE not possible	**Biomarker** **1. Meconium** **Koren G,** et al.Ther Drug Monit 2002; 24 (1):23–25. **Moore C,** et al. Clin Chem 2003; 49 (1):133–136. **Gareri J** et al. Ther Drug Monit 2008; 30 (2):239–245. **Hutson J. R.** et al. Can J Clin Pharm 2007; 14 (2):e169. **Goh, Y. I.,**et al. Clin Pharm Ther 2008; 83 (S1):S75. **2. Hair**

Studientyp/ Autoren, Jahr	Suchstrategie Ein- und Ausschlusskriterien	Welche Behandlungen wurden geprüft	Charakteristik eingeschlossener Studien/Befunde in Bezug auf Diagnostik	Methodische Besonderheiten/ Bemerkungen	Evidenzgraduierung nach CEBM 2009 (University of Oxford)	Literaturbelege
			natal ethanol exposure in the second and third trimester of pregnancy. **Moreover, there has not yet been a correlation of how much FAEE correspond to the development of FASD.** **2. Hair** FAEE have been demonstrated to concentrate in the hair matrix in adults. Studies in neonates have demonstrated that babies exposed to alcohol have been able to quantify FAEE in infants exposed to excessive quantities of alcohol **This test is in its developmental stages and its clinical sensitivity and specificity have not yet been determined.** **3. Cord blood** Gallot et al. measured AST, ALT, GGT, CDT in fetal cord blood to exposed neonates immediately after birth over a 1-year period. Of 870 samples, only 2 cases of FASD were identified and there were no significant correlations between			**Caprara D** L et al. Ther Drug Monit 2005; 27 (6):811–815. **Klein J** et al. Ther Drug Monit 1999; 21 (6):644–646. **3. Cord blood** **Gallot D** et al. Clin Chem Lab Med 2007; 45(4):546–548.

Anhang 4

Studientyp/ Autoren, Jahr	Suchstrategie Ein- und Ausschlusskriterien	Welche Behandlungen wurden geprüft	Charakteristik eingeschlossener Studien/Befunde in Bezug auf Diagnostik	Methodische Besonderheiten/ Bemerkungen	Evidenzgraduierung nach CEBM 2009 (University of Oxford)	Literaturbelege
			maternal and cord blood biomarkers. **Thus, using these parameters is not an effective means of screening for prenatal alcohol exposure.**			

FAS – Faciale Auffälligkeiten

Studientyp/ Autoren, Jahr	Suchstrategie Ein- und Ausschlusskriterien	Welche Behandlungen wurden geprüft	Charakteristik eingeschlossener Studien/Befunde in Bezug auf Diagnostik	Methodische Besonderheiten/ Bemerkungen	Evidenzgraduierung nach CEBM 2009 (University of Oxford)	Literaturbelege
Abdelrahman A et al., 2009 [1] Review with systematic search	Search was conducted in Medline from its inception to March 2009 for original research and review articles relating to prenatal alcohol exposure, using combinations of the terms 'fetal alcohol', 'eye', 'ophthalmic' and 'alcohol teratogenesis'. No language restrictions were applied. Reference lists of identified articles were also searched. Inclusion/Exclusion:	Objective of the review was to describe the effects of prenatal alcohol exposure on the eye, quantify their incidence and comment on their importance in diagnosis of children with FAS.	1) **Short palpebral fissures:** A shortened distance between the inner and outer corners of each eye, defined as a length two or more standard deviations below the mean. The presence of short palpebral fissures is of particular discriminant value in FAS. 2) **Epicanthus:** This is a lateral extension of the skin of the bridge of the nose over the endocanthion. A study found 80 % of children prenatally exposed to ethanol had epicanthus; 3) **Ocular hypertelorism:** Defined as an increased interorbital distance, and may be measured as the distance from right endocanthion to	References are partially not indicated. Quality/methodology of single studies is not described. There is no description of efforts to identify publication bias. How many reviewers the studies assessed is not mentioned. Heterogenity is not discussed.	As quality and design of studies are not indicated a level of evidence (LoE) cannot be assigned or is Expertopinion	1) Clarren SK, Smith DW. New Engl J Med 1978;298(19):1063–7. 2) Manning MA, Hoyme HH. Neurosci Biobehav Rev 2007;31 (2): 230–8. 3) Astley SJ, Clarren SK. Alcohol Alcohol 2001;36(2):147–59. 5) +6) Strömland K. Surv Ophthalmol 1987;31 (4):277. 8) Ribeiro IM et al.. Eur J Ophthalmol 2007;17(1):104–9. Flanigan EY et al.. J Pediatr 2008;153

Studientyp/ Autoren, Jahr	Suchstrategie Ein- und Ausschlusskriterien	Welche Behandlungen wurden geprüft	Charakteristik eingeschlossener Studien/Befunde in Bezug auf Diagnostik	Methodische Besonderheiten/ Bemerkungen	Evidenzgraduierung nach CEBM 2009 (University of Oxford)	Literaturbelege
	detailed criteria not described Patient population: children with FAS		left endocanthion. It is a commonly reported finding in FAS, although not pathognomonic of the condition **4) Coloboma:** Normally the choroid fissure closes during the seventh week of development – failure of closure results in the formation of a distinctive cleft in the iris known as coloboma iridis. This is one of the key extensive malformations that may be found in children with FAS (no reference indicated) **5) Strabismus:** An abnormal alignment of the two eyes. While it is a non-specific finding, it is common in FAS and may be diagnostically useful in conjunction with other features; Strömland et al. found that of thirty children with FAS, 13 had strabismus, 12 of which had a horizontal convergent form (esotropia) **6) Blepharoptosis:** (or ptosis), is drooping of the upper eyelid.	P values, confidence intervals or other statistical measures are not reported.		(3):391–5. Hug TE et al. J Appos 2000;4(4):200–4.

Anhang 4

Studien-typ/ Autoren, Jahr	Suchstrategie Ein- und usschlusskriterien,	Welche Behandlungen wurden geprüft	Charakteristik eingeschlossener Studien/Befunde in Bezug auf Diagnostik	Methodische Besonderheiten/ Bemerkungen	Evidenz-graduierung nach CEBM 2009 (University of Oxford)	Literaturbelege
			Although it is a non-specific sign, Strömland found that 20 % of children with FAS had blepharoptosis. 7) **Microphthalmia:** An abnormally small eye – is a frequent finding in FAS and was included in the Fetal Alcohol Study Group diagnostic criteria. However, the diagnostic usefulness of this condition is limited by difficulty in detection, particularly in the presence of confounding factors such as microcephaly and short palpebral fissures (no reference indicated) 8) **Abnormalities** of the fundus: The fundus may be affected by various abnormalities – the most common findings are hypoplasia of the optic nerve and increased tortuosity of the retinal vessels. In a cohort of Swedish children with FAS, Strömland found optic nerve hypoplasia in 48 % and increased tortuosity in 49 % 2. More recently, Hug et al			

Studientyp/ Autoren, Jahr	Suchstrategie Ein- und Ausschlusskriterien	Welche Behandlungen wurden geprüft	Charakteristik eingeschlossener Studien/Befunde in Bezug auf Diagnostik	Methodische Besonderheiten/ Bemerkungen	Evidenzgraduierung nach CEBM 2009 (University of Oxford)	Literaturbelege
			suggested that prenatal alcohol exposure leads to disturbed retinal function on the basis of abnormal electroretinograms in ten children with FAS. On the whole, the authors recommend • Inspection for periocular features, possibly supplemented by morphometric analysis • Measurement of visual acuity (using visual evoked potentials), visual fields and eye movements • Slit lamp examination of anterior segment and media • Ophthalmoscopic examination with particular attention paid to the optic disc			
Goh I.Y. et al. 2008 Systematic Review Here extracted: underlying	Search Methods: Search in Medline and Pubmed 1966 up to 12/2007 No language restriction Search terms: screen-	Different Screening methods for FAS Evaluation of Test accuracy: Sensitivity Specificity Positive predictive Value	**1. Physical Screening Tools** **1a. Facial Phenotype** *Astley + Clarren 1995*: quantitative case definition of FAS facial phenotype evaluating children 0–10y, 1993–95 Best discriminating between FAS	No consistent information about underlying study quality. Case-Control-Studies	Keine Angabe der Studienqualität – LOE nicht möglich	**1. Physical Screening tools** **1a. Facial Phenotype** Astley SJ, Clarren SK. Alcohol Clin Exp Res 1995; 19 (6):1565–1571.

Anhang 4

Anhang 4

Studientyp/ Autoren, Jahr	Suchstrategie Ein- und Ausschlusskriterien	Welche Behandlungen wurden geprüft	Charakteristik eingeschlossener Studien/Befunde in Bezug auf Diagnostik	Methodische Besonderheiten/ Bemerkungen	Evidenzgraduierung nach CEBM 2009 (University of Oxford)	Literaturbelege
evidence report of the sited publication given in a link [35]	ing, fetal alcohol spectrum disorder, fetal alcohol syndrome Inclusion criteria: methodologies of screening for FASD in children up to 18 years, Studies of adults excluded	Negative predictive Value	and No-Fas: **Hypoplastic midface, smooth philtrum, thin upper lip** **D-scores:** **100 % sensitive,** **87.2 % specific** (3-point Likert scale). *Astley+Clarren 1996* **Development of a photographic screening tool for the FAS facial phenotype** (4-digit diagnostic code: growth deficiency, FAS face phenotype, CNS damage/dysfunction, and gestational alcohol exposure and D-score to measure the magnitude of expression of FAS facial phenotype.	Cohortstudies No information about control groups resp. how the diagnosis was validated		Astley SJ, Clarren SK. J Pediatr 1996; 129 (1):33–41. Astley SJ, Clarren SK. Alcohol Alcohol 2000; 35(4):400–410. Astley SJ et al. J Pediatr 2002; 141 (5):712–717. Avner M, et al. J FAS Int 2006; 4(e20):1–7. Douglas TS, Viljoen DL Ann Hum Biol 2006; 33(2):241–254. Moore ES et al. Alcohol Clin Exp Res 2007; 31 (10):1707–1713. Mutsvangwa T, Douglas TS. J Anat 2007; 210(2):209–220. **1b. Screning Checklist Burd L et al. The FAS Screen**, Addict Biol 1999; 4:329–336. Poitra BA et al. Neu-
Facial			**Evaluation** 1. 42 subjects with FAS/84 controls. Photographs were obtained aligned to the frontal plane and phenotypic expressions were recorded on a 5-point Likert scale. **99 % sensitivity,** **95 % specificity, and** **98 % accuracy.** Sensitivity and specificity were not			

Studien-typ/ Autoren, Jahr	Suchstrategie Ein- und Ausschlusskriterien	Welche Behandlungen wurden geprüft	Charakteristik eingeschlossener Studien/Befunde in Bezug auf Diagnostik	Methodische Besonderheiten/ Bemerkungen	Evidenz-graduierung nach CEBM 2009 (University of Oxford)	Literaturbelege
			affected by race, gender, and age. **2. Astley et al. 2002** Screening of children in a Foster program, age 0–12 years (1999–2001). Facial features were ranked using the Lip-Philtrum Guide in their Fetal Alcohol Syndrome Facial Photographic Analysis Software (Version 1.0.0.). Prevalence of FAS 10/1000. screening tool: **100 % sensitivity, 99.8 % specificity.** 85.7 % predictive value positive, 100 % predictive value negative 3. Validation in 40 children resulted in 4 false positive and no false negative **100 % Sensitivity 64 % Specificity** Problem computer-assisted measurement tended to underestimate true length of palpebral fissure e. < 4y children. 4. Studies with different ethnies revealed that ethnical differences			rotoxicol Teratol 2003; 25(6):725–729.

Anhang 4

Studientyp/ Autoren, Jahr	Suchstrategie Ein- und Ausschlusskriterien,	Welche Behandlungen wurden geprüft	Charakteristik eingeschlossener Studien/Befunde in Bezug auf Diagnostik	Methodische Besonderheiten/ Bemerkungen	Evidenzgraduierung nach CEBM 2009 (University of Oxford)	Literaturbelege
			exist (f. e.eye distance measurement different in southafrican children) Reduces size of eye orbit consistent discriminating feature **Checklist FAS-Screen (32.items)** 1. **Checklist** focuses physical parameters but addresses also developmental changes 100 % sensitivity, 94 %specificity, PPV 92 %, Accuracy 94 % 2. **Validation** in kindergarden children Staff received 4hours of training on the screening tool, 10-minute screening by the school after informed consent „normal sample", **1384 children were screened over 9 years, during which 69 (5 %) were positive. After referral 7 (10 %) were found to have FAS or partial FAS.** Diagnose was given in a center, interdisciplinary experts. **100 % sensitivity 95,43 % specific 95 % accurate**			

Studien-typ/ Autoren, Jahr	Suchstrategie Ein- und usschlusskriterien,	Welche Behandlungen wurden geprüft	Charakteristik eingeschlossener Studien/Befunde in Bezug auf Diagnostik	Methodische Besonderheiten/ Bemerkungen	Evidenz-graduierung nach CEBM 2009 (University of Oxford)	Literaturbelege
FAS – ZNS-strukturelle Auffälligkeiten						
Geuze E, 2005;10 (2):160–84. [34]	Literature search Medline Indexed with keywords Hippocampus, volume and MRI English-language, human subject, 423 relevant hits 1988 up to 12/2003	data-driven papers on hippocampal volumetry	Disease related changes of hippocampus volume	Only results for FAS, Autism, Low birth weight, ADHD stated 1. FAS: 1 study volume not changed compared to controls Archibald SL et al. 2001 14 FAS, 12 AE + 41 healthy controls 2. ADHD: 1 study volume not changed in comparison to controls Castellanos FX et al. 1996 57 boys with ADHD and 55 healthy matched controls	1. Archibald SL et al. 2001 2. Castellanos FX et al. 1996	

Anhang 4

Studientyp/ Autoren, Jahr	Suchstrategie Ein- und Ausschlusskriterien	Welche Behandlungen wurden geprüft	Charakteristik eingeschlossener Studien/Befunde in Bezug auf Diagnostik	Methodische Besonderheiten/ Bemerkungen	Evidenz-graduierung nach CEBM 2009 (University of Oxford)	Literaturbelege
Goh I.Y. et al. 2008 Systematic Review Here extracted: underlying evidence report of the sited publication given in a link	Search Methods: Search in Medline and Pubmed 1966 up to 12/2007 No language restriction Search terms: screening, fetal alcohol spectrum disorder, fetal alcohol syndrome	Different Screening methods for FAS Evaluation of Test accuracy: Sensitivity Specificity Positive predictive Value Negative predictive Value	**Neuroimaging** **1. Ultrasound** ultrasound screening for small for gestational age has 80–90 % sensitivity, but low specificity – many causing conditions 1 study with small number assessing 18 children 5–6weeks after birth: 50 freeze-frame midsaggital sections. Midline corpus callosum in PAE children with abnormal splenium. Results limited by number **2. EEG** see Review D-Angiulli et al. 2006! **3. Magnetic Resonance Imaging** **a. MRI** MRI studies: persons with FASD: • reduction in size of the cranial vault, – reduced brain size – alteration in size and shape of corpus callosum – displacement of corpus callosum – reduction of basal ganglia size – reduction of cerebellum size – reduction in white matter in			**MRI** **Mattson SN** et al. Alcohol Clin Exp Res 1996; 20(5):810–816. **Mattson SN** et al. Alcohol Clin Exp Res 1992; 16 (5):1001–1003. **Mattson SN,** et al. Neurotoxicol Teratol 1994; 16(3):283–289. **Archibald SL et al.,** Dev Med Child Neurol 2001; 43(3):148–154. **Riikonen RS** et al. Biol Psychiatry 2005; 57 (12):1565–1572. **Sowell ER** et al. Cereb Cortex 2002; 12 (8):856–865. **Riley EP** et al. Alcohol Clin Exp Res 1995; 19 (5):1198–1202. **Hynd GW** et al. J Learn Disabil 1991; 24 (3):141–146. **Bhatara VS,** et al. S D J

Anhang 4

Neuroimaging

Studientyp/ Autoren, Jahr	Suchstrategie Ein- und usschlusskriterien,	Welche Behandlungen wurden geprüft	Charakteristik eingeschlossener Studien/Befunde in Bezug auf Diagnostik	Methodische Besonderheiten/ Bemerkungen	Evidenzgraduierung nach CEBM 2009 (University of Oxford)	Literaturbelege
			cerebrum, – altered corpus callosum, frontal and parietal lobe anomalies, – reduced surface area and volume of cerebellum, – altered frontal-striatal response, – abnormal cortical thickness – reduced volume of basal ganglia. – Greater inferior-middle frontal lobe activity was observed in FASD in children and adults. **b. Magnetic Resonance Spectroskopy** – MRS studies demonstrated altered N-acetylaspartate/choline metabolite ratios in persons affected with FASD compared to controls. **MRI has neither been validated as a screening tool nor has specificity and sensitivity been determined.** **Perhaps MRI may be more effective in the diagnostic process to confirm neurological irregularities.** **Diffusion tensor imaging (DTI)** Microstructural abnormalities have been observed in patients with FAS.			Med 2002; 55 (2):59–62. **Bookstein FL**, et al. Neuroimage 2002; 15 (1):233–251. **Bookstein FL** et al., Teratology 2001; 64 (1):4–32. **Riley EP et al.** Am J Med Genet C Semin Med Genet 2004; 127 (1):35–41. **Mattson SN**, et al.Alcohol Clin Exp Res 1996; 20 (6):1088–1093. **Jones KL**, **Smith DW**.. Lancet 1973; 2 (7836):999–1001. **Clarren SK et al.** J Pediatr 1978; 92 (1):64–67. **Swayze VW**,et al. Pediatrics 1997; 99 (2):232–240. **Riikonen R, et al.** Dev Med Child Neurol

Anhang 4

Anhang 4

Studientyp/ Autoren, Jahr	Suchstrategie Ein- und Ausschlusskriterien	Welche Behandlungen wurden geprüft	Charakteristik eingeschlossener Studien/Befunde in Bezug auf Diagnostik	Methodische Besonderheiten/ Bemerkungen	Evidenzgraduierung nach CEBM 2009 (University of Oxford)	Literaturbelege
			1. Study: DTI to examine corpus callosum in adults with FASD – lower fractional anisotrophy, higher MD in splenium and genu of corpus callosum vs. controls. No associations between DTI and dysmorphia score, IQ or processing speed. 2. Study: 14 children (10–13) trend toward smaller total cerebral volume p = 0,057 vs. controls. Greater mean diffusivity in the isthmus of corpus callosum (p = 0,013). **The disadvantages are the same as MRI**			1999; 41(10):652–659. **Clark CM**, et al. Pediatrics 2000; 105 (5):1096–1099. **Bookstein FL**, et al. Anat Rec 2002; 269 (3):162–174. **Johnson VP** et al. Am J Med Genet 1996; 61 (4):329–339. **Sowell ER**, et al. Neuroreport 2001; 12 (3):515–523. **Fryer SL**, et al. Alcohol Clin Exp Res 2007; 31 (8):1415–1424. **Sowell ER**, et al. Cereb Cortex 2008; 18 (1):136–144. **Malisza KL**, et al. Pediatr Res 2005; 58 (6):1150–1157. <u>MRS</u> **Fagerlund A** et al. Alcohol Clin Exp Res 2006; 30 (12):2097–2104.

Studientyp/ Autoren, Jahr	Suchstrategie Ein- und Ausschlusskriterien,	Welche Behandlungen wurden geprüft	Charakteristik eingeschlossener Studien/Befunde in Bezug auf Diagnostik	Methodische Besonderheiten/ Bemerkungen	Evidenzgraduierung nach CEBM 2009 (University of Oxford)	Literaturbelege
Systematic review/ D'Angiulli et al. 2006 [29]	**Databases:** Systematic search in Medline, reference check **Period** 1966 to June 2006 **Inclusion criterias:** Publication in peer-refereed journal. at least summaries of EEG or evoked potential (EP) data, English publications	**Reseach questions:** 1.) Is EEG a useful neuroimaging technique for investigating the brain correlates of PEA (prenatal alcohol exposure) in infants and children? 2. Are there indeed consistent EEG correlates of PEA in literature? 3.)	17 publications (16 studies) were included. Information on study designs and methodological quality are not given by the authors. The studies were evaluated according to three types of processes that were measured (Sleep and wakefulness, sensory processes, attention). **1. Sleep and wakefulness** 7 Studies (n = 491), 6 analyzed infants, in 1 study participants were 4–19 years. All children were classified as PEA positive. No study used a FAS diagnosis as re-	Review searched only in Medline Methodological quality of studies was not systematically assessed and considered. Publication bias not considered. There is no specific question which structured the re-	4	Cortese BM, et al. Neurotoxicol Teratol 2006; 28(5):597–606. DTI Wozniak JR, Lim KO. Neurosci Biobehav Rev 2006; 30 (6):762–774. Ma X et al. Alcohol Clin Exp Res 2005; 29(7):1214–1222. **Literatur according to the types of processes** **Sleep and wakefulness** Chernick, V., Childiaeva, R., & Ioffe, S. (1983). Am J Obstet Gynecol 146, 41–47. Havlicek et al. Ioffe, S., & Chernick, V. (1988). Dev Med Child Neurol 30, 797–807. Ioffe, S., & Chernick,

Anhang 4

Studientyp/ Autoren, Jahr	Suchstrategie Ein- und ausschlusskriterien,	Welche Behandlungen wurden geprüft	Charakteristik eingeschlossener Studien/Befunde in Bezug auf Diagnostik	Methodische Besonderheiten/ Bemerkungen	Evidenzgraduierung nach CEBM 2009 (University of Oxford)	Literaturbelege
	Patient population infants and children with known prenatal exposure to alcohol (PEA), including Fetal Alcohol Syndrome (FAS) and more subtle but adverse neuroanatomical and neurobehavioral problems, described as fetal alcohol effects (FAE)	On the basis of EEG correlates, are there emerging implications for the study of PEA and its effects in infants and children.	inclusion criteria. **Summary of findings:** EEG studies on the effects of PEA in infants and children specifically focusing on sleep and wakefulness show that different patterns and timing of alcohol consumption by mothers have a differential impact on infants' brain. Patterns of neonatal EEG hypersynchrony and increased spectral power during REM and quiet sleep are consistent correlates of PEA, which are not confounded by the use of other substances. Some evidence also suggests that abnormal EEG activity during sleep in infants is associated with later developmental outcomes.

2. Sensory processes
5 Studies (n = 127), in 3 studies infants were analyzed, 1 study analyzed participants from 0,2 to 17 years, in 1 study age was unknown. 3 studies focused on auditory evoked potential (EP) and 2 studies | view. This is more an overview of available studies.

Most serious limitations of the evidence according to the authors:
1.) Difficulty in comparing studies that used different measures (such as threshold for hearing loss),
2.) insufficient details of methodology (i. e., specific type of EEG anomaly, detailed description of subjects),
3.) highly questionable reliability of assessing alcohol consumption solely by self-reporting methods, | | V. (1990). Neuropediatrics 21, 11–17.
Ioffe et al. (1984). Pediatrics 74, 330–335.
Scher et al. (1988). Pediatr Res 24, 101–105.
O'Malley, K., & Barr, H. (1998). Can J Psychol 43, 1051.

Sensory processes
Church, M., & Gerkin, K. (1988). Pediatrics 82, 147–154.
Pettigrew, A., & Hutchinson, I. (1984). Ciba Found Symp 105, 26–46.
Rossig et al. (1994). Neuropediatrics 25, 245–249.
Scher et al. (1988). Pediatr Res 24, 101–105.
Olegard et al. (1979). Acta Paediatr Scand |

Studien-typ/ Autoren, Jahr	Suchstrategie Ein- und Ausschlusskriterien	Welche Behandlungen wurden geprüft	Charakteristik eingeschlossener Studien/Befunde in Bezug auf Diagnostik	Methodische Besonderheiten/ Bemerkungen	Evidenz-graduierung nach CEBM 2009 (University of Oxford)	Literaturbelege
			on visual and somatosensory EP. 2 studies used a FAS diagnosis as inclusion criteria. **Summary of findings:** all studies focusing on sensory processes in infants and children with PEA have found evidence of sensory impairment suggestive of atypical brain maturation. From these studies, it seems that the cluster of conditions associated with PEA may include impaired hearing, vision, and somatosensory functions that presumably persist through the entire development and life span. **3. Attention and cognition** 4 Studies (n = 75), participants age ranged from 4 to 15 years, all studies used FAS diagnosis as inclusion criteria. **Summary of findings:** EEG and EP studies focusing on attention and cognitive functions have indicated that these techniques can be valuable in providing functional assessment of the brain	often long after the actual event, 4.) lack of control for several factors that influence the exposure of the fetus to alcohol (e. g., critical developmental periods, patterns of exposure, and maternal metabolism).		Suppl 275, 112–121. **Attention and cognition** **Buffington** et al. (1981). Neurobehav Toxicol Teratol 3, 183–185. **Kaneko** et al. (1996a). Alcohol Clin Exp Res 20, 35–42. **Kaneko** et al. (1996b). Clin Neurophysiol 98, 20–28. **Mattson** et al. (1992). Alcohol Clin Exp Res 16, 1001–1003.

Studientyp, Autoren, Jahr	Suchstrategie Ein- und Ausschlusskriterien,	Welche Behandlungen wurden geprüft	Charakteristik eingeschlossener Studien/Befunde in Bezug auf Diagnostik	Methodische Besonderheiten/ Bemerkungen	Evidenzgraduierung nach CEBM 2009 (University of Oxford)	Literaturbelege
			of children with PEA. Although there is no clear marker of specific effects of PEA, the available data suggest that older children may suffer impairments in attention and/or related cognitive functions that are associated. **Concrete Findings:** **Kaneko (n = 18 FAS 4–15y)** 1. Atypical EP (P300) – significant longer wave latencies in FAS vs. Down or Control Children 2. in 50 % of FAS children borderline or abnormal EEG: immature, low amplitude, parietal lobe more affected **Buffington (n = 10 FAS 6–14y, controls)** Reduced or absent contingent negative variation not statistically significant low sample size) **Mattson (n = 2 FAS 13+14y)** Moderately abnormal EEGs; theta activity dominant **Spohr and Steinhausen (n = 45 FSA, 4–8J, Follow up 3–4)** Fewer			

Studientyp/ Autoren, Jahr	Suchstrategie Ein- und Ausschlusskriterien,	Welche Behandlungen wurden geprüft	Charakteristik eingeschlossener Studien/Befunde in Bezug auf Diagnostik	Methodische Besonderheiten/ Bemerkungen	Evidenzgraduierung nach CEBM 2009 (University of Oxford)	Literaturbelege
			abnormal EEGs at follow up! First EEG 51 % normal acticity, Follow up after 3 years 71 % normal Severe Sleep disturbances 22 % follow up 15 %. „Although these children also improved with regard to neurologic performance, psychiatric status, and cognitive function, they continued to show hyperactivity and distractibility at school, and a persisting handicap, particularly reflected in low levels of educational achievement, was evident."			

FAS – dysfunctional behaviour/mental health

Studientyp/ Autoren, Jahr	Suchstrategie Ein- und Ausschlusskriterien,	Welche Behandlungen wurden geprüft	Charakteristik eingeschlossener Studien/Befunde in Bezug auf Diagnostik	Methodische Besonderheiten/ Bemerkungen	Evidenzgraduierung nach CEBM 2009 (University of Oxford)	Literaturbelege
Goh I.Y. et al. 2008 Systematic Review Here extracted: underlying evidence report of	Search Methods: Search in Medline and Pubmed 1966 up to 12/2007 No language restriction Search terms: screening, fetal alcohol spectrum disorder, fetal alcohol syndrome	Different Screening methods for FAS Evaluation of Test accuracy: Sensitivity Specificity Positive predictive Value Negative predictive Value	**Psychological/Neurobehavioural/ Neurophysiological** There is limited literature regarding using psychological evaluations to screen for FASD. The majority of literature reports on psychological testing as a process used in of FASD diagnoses. Testing methods include the use of Bayley Scales, Wechsler Intelligence	Case-control studies,	LoE 3–4	**1. Streissguth AP,** Bookstein FL, Barr HM, Press S, Sampson PD. A fetal alcohol behavior scale. Alcohol Clin Exp Res 1998; 22(2):325–333. **2. Nash K,** et al. Arch Womens Ment Health 2006; 9(4):181–186.

Anhang 4

Studientyp/ Autoren, Jahr	Suchstrategie Ein- und Ausschlusskriterien,	Welche Behandlungen wurden geprüft	Charakteristik eingeschlossener Studien/Befunde in Bezug auf Diagnostik	Methodische Besonderheiten/ Bemerkungen	Evidenzgraduierung nach CEBM 2009 (University of Oxford)	Literaturbelege
the sited publication given in a link **Neuropsych.**	Inclusion criteria: methodologies of screening for FASD in children up to 18 years, Studies of adults excluded		Scale for Children (WISC-III), Griffiths Mental Developmental Scales, Wechsler Preschool and Primary Scale of Intelligence (WPPSI-R), Fagan Test of Infant Intelligence, Children's Memory Scale (CMS), Behavioral Rating Inventory of Executive Function (BRIEF), Parent and Teachers Conners' Ratings Scales-Revised (CRS-R), and Child Behavioral Checklist (CBCL). 1. 36-item scale: the Fetal Alcohol Behavior Scale (FABS), Streissguth et al. Development and Evaluation 5 minute questionnaire. 186 caregivers completed for their children. Cronbach's coefficient: 0.89, indicating high reliability. FABS scores appear to be correlated with maternal alcohol problems and reflect the behavioral phenotype of fetal alcohol fairly specifically rather than being raised in an alcoholic environment.			**Greenbaum R**, et al. Can J Clin Pharmacol 2002; 9(4): 215–225. **3. Green CR, et al.** Alcohol Clin Exp Res 2007; 31(3):500–511. **4a. Green JH.** J Sch Health 2007; 77 (3):103–108. **4b. Kodituwakku PW** et al, Alcohol Clin Exp Res 1995; 19 (6):1558–1564. **Mattson SN**, Riley EP. J Int Neuropsychol Soc 1999; 5(5):462–471. **Schonfeld AM** et al, J Stud Alcohol 2001; 62 (2):239–246. **4c. Olson HC,** et al, Semin Clin Neuropsychiatry 1998; 3 (4):262–284. **Burd L,** et al, Neurotoxicol Teratol 2003; 25 (6):697–705.

Studientyp/ Autoren, Jahr	Suchstrategie Ein- und Ausschlusskriterien	Welche Behandlungen wurden geprüft	Charakteristik eingeschlossener Studien/Befunde in Bezug auf Diagnostik	Methodische Besonderheiten/ Bemerkungen	Evidenzgraduierung nach CEBM 2009 (University of Oxford)	Literaturbelege
			Further studies are needed to clarify its utility in a diagnosis or screening context. Instruments like the FABS should not be used clinically for diagnosis without additional evidence of prenatal alcohol exposure. **2. CBCL** The CBCL has open-ended questions and a rating scale of 113 behavioural descriptors Greenbaum et al: CBCL in a sample of 35 children affected with ARND. Significant differences in 62 items when compared to a control group of 35 matched for age, gender, and socioeconomic status. **Twelve items were significantly different p < 0.00 196.** These were 'acts too young for age', 'argues', 'can't concentrate=poor attention', 'can't sit still=restless=hyperactive', 'cruelty, bullying or meanness to others', 'disobedient at home', 'no guilt after misbehaving', 'impulsive=acts without			**Steinhausen HC**, Spohr HL.. Alcohol Clin Exp Res 1998; 22 (2):334–338.82 **4 d. Kodituwakku PW** et al, Alcohol Clin Exp Res 1995; 19 (6):1558–1564. **Mattson SN**, Riley EP. Alcohol Clin Exp Res 2000; 24(2):226–231. **Coles CD**, et al, Alcohol Clin Exp Res 1997; 21(1):150–161. **4 e. Streissguth AP**, et al, Psychol Sci 1999; 10 (3):186–190. **Mattson SN**, Riley EP. Alcohol Clin Exp Res 1998; 22(2):279–294. **Olson HC**, et al, J Am Acad Child Adolesc Psychiatry 1997; 36(9):1187–1194.

Studientyp/ Autoren, Jahr	Suchstrategie Ein- und Ausschlusskriterien,	Welche Behandlungen wurden geprüft	Charakteristik eingeschlossener Studien/Befunde in Bezug auf Diagnostik	Methodische Besonderheiten/ Bemerkungen	Evidenzgraduierung nach CEBM 2009 (University of Oxford)	Literaturbelege
			thinking', 'lying or cheating', 'showing off=clowning', 'steals from home', and 'steals outside' Nash et al.: Evaluation with a sample of children diagnosed with FASD and ADHD. Parents of 54 children (11 FAS, 43 ARND) completed the CBCL. In this study the 12 items were scored. **Seven of the 12 items strongly differentiated FASD children from ADHD and normal controls (p < 0001).** They were "no guilt", "lying or cheating", "can't concentrate", "restless", "impulsive", "disobedient", and "acts young". Six items differentiated the FAS/ ARND from ADHD group (P<0001). They were "no guilt", "cruelty", "acts young", "steals from home", "steals outside", and "lying or cheating". **86 % sensitivity and 82 % specificity were observed with 6 of the 7 items when comparing FASD, ADHD, and controls.**			

Studien-typ/ Autoren, Jahr	Suchstrategie Ein- und Ausschlusskriterien,	Welche Behandlungen wurden geprüft	Charakteristik eingeschlossener Studien/Befunde in Bezug auf Diagnostik	Methodische Besonderheiten/ Bemerkungen	Evidenz-graduierung nach CEBM 2009 (University of Oxford)	Literaturbelege
			81 % sensitivity and 72 % specificity were observed with 3 of 6 items when comparing FASD vs. ADHD group („no guilt", „cruelty", „acts young"). From these observations Nash et al. proposed that a FASD screening tool should be considered involving a 2-step approach: first identify behaviours suggesting FASD and then discriminate FASD from ADHD. The limitation is that these are primary results which have not been replicated in a large sample size. In addition it has not been validated in different ethnicities or languages. **3. Ocular motor testing.** Ocular motor tasks are sensitive tools for assesing executive function. Green et al. measured saccadic reaction times in FASD and control children 8–12 years 97. Children with FASD were observed to have elongated reaction times, excessive direction error, and no			

Anhang 4

Studien-typ/ Autoren, Jahr	Suchstrategie Ein- und usschlusskriterien,	Welche Behandlungen wurden geprüft	Charakteristik eingeschlossener Studien/Befunde in Bezug auf Diagnostik	Methodische Besonderheiten/ Bemerkungen	Evidenz-graduierung nach CEBM 2009 (University of Oxford)	Literaturbelege
			express saccades compared to controls. This tool is very early in its development and further investigation is warranted to establish its validity and reproducibility. **4. Range of Studies on neuropsychological issues:** a. **Persons affected with FASD** have deficits in cognitive and academic functioning, psychological disorders behavioural problems, and difficulties with independent living. b. **Neuropsychological sequelae** including executive functioning difficulties have been observed. c. **Social skills deficits** including poor social judgment, failure to learn from experience, difficulty understanding consequences of actions, aggression, inappropriate sexual behaviour, delinquency, lack of understanding of social cues, and communicating in social contexts have also been observed. Individuals with FASD also often de-			

Studien-typ/ Autoren, Jahr	Suchstrategie Ein- und Ausschlusskriterien,	Welche Behandlungen wurden geprüft	Charakteristik eingeschlossener Studien/Befunde in Bezug auf Diagnostik	Methodische Besonderheiten/ Bemerkungen	Evidenz-graduierung nach CEBM 2009 (University of Oxford)	Literaturbelege
			monstrate impulsivity, poor judgment, and great difficulty learning from consequences. **d. Hyperactivity and attention problems** are some of the **most frequently reported** symptoms associated with prenatal alcohol exposure and reported in the research literature. **e.** Exposure to alcohol in the first and second trimesters has been associated with **lower overall academic achievement.** Lower reading scores, spatial and verbal memory and learning were associated with second trimester binge drinking as were problems in processing and arithmetic. Mattson et al. reviewed IQ in many studies with **children diagnosed with FAS and found a mean of 65.73 (20–120). The mean IQ for FASD was 72.26 (47.4–98.2)** They concluded that high levels of prenatal alcohol exposure are re-			

Anhang 4

Studientyp/ Autoren, Jahr	Suchstrategie Ein- und Ausschlusskriterien	Welche Behandlungen wurden geprüft	Charakteristik eingeschlossener Studien/Befunde in Bezug auf Diagnostik	Methodische Besonderheiten/ Bemerkungen	Evidenzgraduierung nach CEBM 2009 (University of Oxford)	Literaturbelege
Momino W. et al. 2008 Review with systematic search [44]	Literature search in Pubmed between 1968 and 2006 search terms ethanol, pregnancy, behaviour limits: human no information about number of hits or inclusion criteria	Focus on literature on FAS adressing maladaptive behaviour	lated to increased eficits in intellectual functioning. Contents of included studies with children/youth: **1. + 2. Streissguth et al. 1996 and 1997** 415 patients with FAS or FASD a. experience of mental health problem > 90 % b. disrupted school 60 % c. trouble with law 60 %, 32 % incarcerated for a crime d. confinement 50 %, e. inappropriate sexual behaviour 50 % f. alcohol/drug problem 30 % **protective factors (only the first 4)** a. longer period of living in a stable and nuturant home b. being diagnosed with FAS or FASD before the age of 6 years c. never experienced violence against oneself d. longer duration of resicende in each living **3. Boland et al. 1998**	no information about number of hits or inclusion criteria No characteristic of included studies, only communication of content.	4–5	**1. Streissguth AP et al**, (CDC). Seattle: University of Washington, Fetal Alcohol & Drug Unit; 1996. **2. Streissguth AP.** Seattle: University of Washington Press; 1997. p. 25–39. **3. Boland FJ.** Correctional Service of Canada; 1998. **4. Fast DK**, Conry J, Loock CA. 1999;20:370–2. **5. Conry J**, Fast DK. British Columbia Fetal Alcohol Syndrome Resource Society; 2000.

Studien-typ/ Autoren, Jahr	Suchstrategie Ein- und Ausschlusskriterien,	Welche Behandlungen wurden geprüft	Charakteristik eingeschlossener Studien/Befunde in Bezug auf Diagnostik	Methodische Besonderheiten/ Bemerkungen	Evidenz-graduierung nach CEBM 2009 (University of Oxford)	Literaturbelege
Pei J. et al. 2011 Systematic review [54]	Search in Medline, PsycINFO, Google Scholar, Academic Search Complete and Education Resources Information Centre Search terms FASD, ARND, FAS PAE paired with mental health, depression, oppositional defiant disorder	Prevalence and scope of mental health issues 1. Mental health in childhood and adolescents 2. FASD and mood and anxiety disorders 3. FASD and Attention deficit hyperactivity disorder (ADHD) 4. FASD and CD	1. **Mental health in childhood and adolescence** **Cohort study:** Steinhausen and Spohr 1998: 158 West German children followed from preschool til adolescence 1977–1991 – cognitive impairments and psychiatric symptoms are generally persistent. 63 % of sample with diagnose of at least 1 psychiatric disorder. High rates of psychopathology developmental pathway similar to similar to attention deficit disorder (ADD) with or without hyperactivity Predictors of conduct disorder similar: Impulsivity, low intelligence, poor school achievement, antisocial behaviour 4.+5. **FAST et al. 1999, Conry et al. 2000** Prevalence of FASD in youth in the criminal systems 287 offenders 23,3 % 67 with alcohol related diagnosis, 3 with FAS diagnosed before	No flow chart of search given (hits, numbers of excluded studies) No inclusion criteria given		**Steinhausen HC** et al. (1998), Alcoholism: Clinical and experimental Research, 22,334–338 **Fryer S.** et al. (2007), Pediatrics,119, e733–741 **Walthall J.** et al 2008. Mental health Aspects of Developmental

Anhang 4

Anhang 4

Studientyp/ Autoren, Jahr	Suchstrategie Ein- und Ausschlusskriterien,	Welche Behandlungen wurden geprüft	Charakteristik eingeschlossener Studien/Befunde in Bezug auf Diagnostik	Methodische Besonderheiten/ Bemerkungen	Evidenzgraduierung nach CEBM 2009 (University of Oxford)	Literaturbelege
	(ODD), conduct disorder (CD) and anxiety disorder	(other outcomes not reported in this table)	(hyperkinetic, emotional. conduct, sleep disorders, sterotypies, abnormal habits) **Case-control Fryer 2007**: 39 American children (12,11) matched to 30 nonalcohol-exposed children (11,2.l) for age, gender, SES. Stand. Diagn. And Statistical Manual of Mental Disorders-IV with all caregivers 97,44 % with at least one Axis I disorder vs. 40 % of nonalcohol-exposed controls. Sign. Diff. (p < 0,05) in ADHD, depressive disorder, oppositional defiant disorder, conduct disorder, anxiety disorder,. 71,5 % vs 50 % disruptive disorders **Case series O'Connor et al. 2006**: 130 patients from an inpatient psychiatric setting in the US, 30 % prenatal alcohol exposed (m.a. 8.64), 7,7 % met criteris for FAS 2. FAS and mood and anxiety disorders **Case-Control Fryer 2007**: FAS-Chil-			Disabilities, 11, 69–78 **Streissguth AP** et al., 1996, Seattle: University of Washington, Fetal Alcohol and Drug unit. Disney E et al 2008, Pediatrics, 122, 1225–1230. **Schonefeld AM** et al. 2005,Journal of studies onj alcohol, 66, 545–554 **Barr HM et al.**, 2006, American Journal of Psychiatry, 163,1061–1065 **Clark et al. 2004**, Journal of Fetal Alcohol Syndrom International.2, 1–12 **Yates et al., 1998**, Alcoholism: Clinical and Experimental Research,22, 914–920 **O'Connor** MJ et al. 2006, Mental Health

Studien-typ/ Autoren, Jahr	Suchstrategie Ein- und Ausschlusskriterien,	Welche Behandlungen wurden geprüft	Charakteristik eingeschlossener Studien/Befunde in Bezug auf Diagnostik	Methodische Besonderheiten/ Bemerkungen	Evidenz-graduierung nach CEBM 2009 (University of Oxford)	Literaturbelege
			dren with more internalizing disorders then general population Case series O'Connor et al. 2002: 23 american in- and outpatient children (5–13J) 87 % with psychiatric disorder, 61 % of which were mood disorders Walthall et al. 2008 link between anxiety, mood disorders, and PAE **3. FAS and ADHD** **Mattson et al, 2006:** significant attention problems among children and adolescents with FAS. **Cohortstudy Streissguth et al. 1996** n = 415 6–51J, mean 14J 60 % attention related problems reported by caretakers **Case-Control Study Fryer 2007**: FAS with 95 % ADHD, controls with 30 % p < 0,05 **Case-Control Study Coles et al. 1997** n = 149 low-income 7–8.5J African American children (mean 7.63) 4 groups Only ADHD = greatest difficulty			Aspects of Developmental Disabilities, 9, 105–109. **O'Connor MJ** et al. 2006. Journal of Pediatric Psychology, 31 (1), 50–64. **Mattson SN** et al., 2006. Neuropsychology, 20, 361–369. **Coles CD** et al., 1997. Alcoholism: Clinical and Experimental Research, 21, 150–161. **Burden MJ** et al., 2005 Alcoholism: Clinical and Experimental Research, 29 (3), 443–452. **O'Malley KD and Nanson J**., 2002. Canadian Journal of Psychiatry, 47, 349–354. **Disney et al. 2008**

Anhang 4

Studientyp/ Autoren, Jahr	Suchstrategie Ein- und Ausschlusskriterien,	Welche Behandlungen wurden geprüft	Charakteristik eingeschlossener Studien/Befunde in Bezug auf Diagnostik	Methodische Besonderheiten/ Bemerkungen	Evidenzgraduierung nach CEBM 2009 (University of Oxford)	Literaturbelege
			with focused and sustained attention FAS = deficits in visual/spatial skills, encoding of the information they focused on, flexibility in problem solving. **Case serie Burden et al. 2005:** 337 African-American children 7,5J prospectively recuited to overrepresent PAE moderate to heavy level no evidence of sustained attention deficits Most affected: working memory ability to actively manipulate information in memory-related task execution Only ADHD specific problems in response inhibition. **Review O'Malley and Nanson (2002):** children with FAS and ADHD comorbidities unique in the ADHD presentation **Bhatara et al. 2006:** A review of 2231 charts of children with PAE (mean age 8,7) found ADHD as most prevalent disorder			

Studientyp/ Autoren, Jahr	Suchstrategie Ein- und usschlusskriterien,	Welche Behandlungen wurden geprüft	Charakteristik eingeschlossener Studien/Befunde in Bezug auf Diagnostik	Methodische Besonderheiten/ Bemerkungen	Evidenzgraduierung nach CEBM 2009 (University of Oxford)	Literaturbelege
			4. FAS and Conduct Disorder Two cohort studies (not matched for IQ) showed that PAE (FU at 17 years) was significantly associated with CD (Disney et al 2008, Schoenefeld et al 2005). Only Schoenefeld et al included children with FAS. The children with FAS did'nt show conduct disorder.			

FAS – Birth defects Liver, Kidney, GI

| Hofer R, Burd L. Clin Mol Teratol 2009;85 (3):179–83. [37] Systematic Review | Search in Pubmed Terms: fetal alcohol syndrome and gastrointestinal tract, liver, kidney, congenital abnormalities „all years" no end of search stated, only English citations only studies with evidence of examination of subjects for FASD (FAS, fetalalcohol effect, alcohol embryopathy, partial FAS or FASD) and specifying | Studies of
1. liver
2. kidney
3. gastrointestinal birth defects in fetal alcohol spectrum disorders | **No distinctive abnormality associated with FASD for either of the three organ systems was found**
1. n = 12 publications of co-occurence of birth defects of the liver and FASD
19 case reports
14 newborns up to 1 year, 5 1 y up to 8 years
n = 7 hyperbilirubinemia, raised liverenzymes
n = 3 hepatomegaly with fibrosis (Birth, 4 Month, 17 Month)
single cases with vascuolar degenerative changes (4y), fatty degen- | | case reports, 1 case serie | **1. Co-occurence of liver birth defects**
Dunigan and Werlin 1981
Habbick et al. 1979
Mooller et al. 1979
Newman et al. 1979
Peiffer et al. 1979
Christoffel and salafsky, 1975
Jones and Smith 1973
Khan et al. 1979
Mulvihil et al. 1976
Lefkowitch et al. 1983
Rosenlicht et al. 1979
Van Dyke et al. 1982 |

Anhang 4

Studientyp/ Autoren, Jahr	Suchstrategie Ein- und usschlusskriterien,	Welche Behandlungen wurden geprüft	Charakteristik eingeschlossener Studien/Befunde in Bezug auf Diagnostik	Methodische Besonderheiten/ Bemerkungen	Evidenzgraduierung nach CEBM 2009 (University of Oxford)	Literaturbelege
	an association between FASD and abnormalities only humans + hand searching of reference lists		eration (5y), Hepatoblastoma (27 Months) etc. 2. n = 12 publications of co-occurrence of birth defects of the kidney and FASD 27 case report, 1 case serie (n = 76) n = 4 Hydronephrosis, n = 9 renal hypoplasy n = 14 single other causes Case serie: „minimal renal findings" 3. n = 2 publications of co-occurrence of gastrointestinal birth defects and FASD 7 case reports n = 5 with chronic intestinal pseudoobstruction in children aged 20 months to 9 years n = 2 (twins) with gastroschisis in both twins			**2. Co-occurence of kidney birth defects** Tenbrinck et Buchin, 1975 Hanson et al. 1978 Goetzman et al. 1975 DeBeukelar and Rndall 1977 Dunigan and Werlin 1981 Havers et al. 1980 Qazi et al. 1979 Sokol et al. 1980 Smith et al. 1981 Mulvihill et al. 1976 Assadi 1990 Goldstein and Arulanantham 1978 **3. Co-occurence of gastrointestinal birth defects** Uc A. et al. 1997 Sarda P., Barth H, 1984

Tab. 2: Evidenztabelle zu funktionellen ZNS-Auffälligkeiten

Publikation (Autor, Jahr) Studientyp	Anzahl der Patienten Patientenmerkmale	Diagnostische Intervention/ Referenzstandard	Outcomes	Ergebnisse	Bemerkungen	Evidenzklassifikation nach Oxford
Neuropsychological Profile/Diagnostic Tools in general						
Astley S.J. et al. 2006 [9] USA, Washington	n = 952 with Evaluation for FAS, 16 with confirmed absence of prenatal alcohol exposure	Comparison of the 4 diagnostic digit code and the Hoyme fetal alcohol spectrum disorders guidelines Hoyme: only 2 from 3 facial criteria in comparison to 4DDC, using 10th percentile, 4DDC using 3 criteria, and < 3th percentile as cut-off for philtrum microcephaly and growth retardation measures	Prevalence of diagnosis FAS with eather test	1. 3,7 % FAS with 4 Diagnostic Digit Code (n = 35) 2. 4,1 % FAS with Hoyme Guidelines (n = 39) Only 17 Patients similar! 35% of patients with Hoyme facial criteria positive (n = 330), low specificity! Only 39 met alle Hoyme FAS criteria 4/16 children without alcohol exposure were positive fo Hoyme Facial criteria **Hoyme exclude functional and neurologic measures of CNS, only include structural, morphologic measures** **Conclusion of the author:** Without a specific facial phenotype, a valid diagnosis of fetal alcohol syndrome cannot be rendered for patients with prenatal alcohol exposure, because a causal	Hoyme does not seem to be adequate for diagnosing FAS 4DDC –good refererence standard?	4

Anhang 4

Publikation (Autor, Jahr) Studientyp	Anzahl der Patienten Patientenmerkmale	Diagnostische Intervention/ Referenzstandard	Outcomes	Ergebnisse	Bemerkungen	Evidenzklassifikation nach Oxford
				link between their outcomes and exposure cannot be established, and a valid diagnosis of fetal alcohol syndrome cannot be rendered for patients with unknown alcohol exposure, because the face cannot serve as a valid proxy measure for alcohol exposure. Diagnostic guidelines must confirm the specificity of their fetal alcohol syndrome facial criteria to validate their diagnostic criteria.		
Aragon AS et al. Alcohol Clin Exp Res 2008;32 (11):1909–19 [2] Case- Control-Study Italy	n = 80 children 6–7 years n = 23 with FAS (19 partial FAS) according to revised IOM criteria (Hoyme 2005) n = 57 peer controls actively randomly assigned from the same 1st grade cohort same classes informed consent of the par-	Tests done by italian licensed psychologists affiliated with the University of Rome blinded to the membership of children 3 h test battery Mothers+ Teachers: Parent/Teacher Disruptive Behaviour Disorder Rating Scale (Pelham	Differences (SD) In 1. Disruptive behaviour focussing on inattention and hyperactivity/ impulsivity 2. Verbal. performance and Fullscale IQ WISC-R profile analysis on 12 subtests	1. Teacher Disruptive Behaviour rating of attention sign. higher for FAS p = 0,05. Hyperactivity/Impulsivity similar. Parent ratings not sign. 2. FAS with significant lower scores on Verbal IQ 0,015, Performance IQ p < 0,01, Full Scale IQ p = 0,01 WISCR-profile analysis sign.	Main limitations: IQ was not a covariate, – possible impact on findings. Limited generalzability due to small sample size.	4

Publikation (Autor, Jahr) Studientyp	Anzahl der Patienten Patientenmerkmale	Diagnostische Intervention/ Referenzstandard	Outcomes	Ergebnisse	Bemerkungen	Evidenzklassifikation nach Oxford
	ents all children of 25 schools randomly selected out of 68 elementary schools close to Rome, Laszio Region (spanning 60 km) Mothers did not differ significantly in age, education, income FAS-children age + gender well matched to controls Significantly differences in: Height, centile, weight, head circumference, total dysmorphology score	1992) Only items for assessing inattention and hyperactivity/impulsivity + Italian Questionnaire to identify difficulties in Learning) Test used: **Wechsler Intelligence Scale for Children Revised** (WISC-R;Rubini&-Padovani 1986) valid Italian Version **Rustioni-Test** (1994, Italian specific normed linguistic understanding, modelled after Test for Reception of Grammar Bishop 1989 **IPDA questionnaire** (Terrini 2002) to measure academic achievement in language and math Italian normed **Raven Colored Progressive Matrices (CPM)** to assess nonverbal rea-	information, similarities, arithmetic, vocabulary, comprehension, memory, picture completion, picture arrangement. Block design, object assembly, coding and mazes. (MANOVA) 3. Language comprehension 4. Nonverbal Intelligence 5. Discriminative function of differences 6. Correlation with FAS features	Deviated from parallelism for FAS. FAS scored sign. lower especially for Block design ($p = 0,02$, object assembly $p < 0,01$ and Mazes $p = 0,03$. Similarity and Vocabulary similar. IQ Scores FAS fell within the average range 3.+4. Almost all Raven CPM (incl. percentile score) $p = 0,007$ and $0,015$ lower for FAS = nonverbal abstract reasoning. Rustioni (qualitative language understanding) $p = 0,028$ lower for FAS only similar for errors made IPDA $p = 0,05$ lower for FAS = academic achievement 5. Teacher rating of attention and hyperactiviy = X^2 12,16 $p = 0,002$, accounted		

Anhang 4

Publikation (Autor, Jahr) Studientyp	Anzahl der Patienten Patientenmerkmale	Diagnostische Intervention/ Referenzstandard	Outcomes	Ergebnisse	Bemerkungen	Evidenzklassifikation nach Oxford
		soning ability Alderton&Larson 1990. **Mothers:** collection of epidemiological data Demographic variables, **drinking patterns.** Nutrition, fertility, childbearing, behaviourial health issues Interview by employees of the University of Rome		for 15 % of the between group variability and maximally separated FASD-Diagnosed children from controls 75 % correct classified. Attentional problems 73,9 % of children correct classified – Best discriminator according to loading matrix FAS more inattentivs symptoms 26 % vs 5 % controls P=0,08 similar rate of hyperactivity 6. Pearson product correlation coefficients between height, weight and head circumference centiles, Total Dysmorphology Raw Score, FullScale, Verbal and performance IQ Scores and Raven CPM percentile scores: Head circumference high correlated with WISC-R summary score as was dys-		

Publikation (Autor, Jahr) Studientyp	Anzahl der Patienten Patientenmerkmale	Diagnostische Intervention/ Referenzstandard	Outcomes	Ergebnisse	Bemerkungen	Evidenzklassifikation nach Oxford
Astley SJ et al. The Can J Clin Pharmacol **2009**;16:e178-e201. [11] Case-Control-Study	N = 81 children, Age 8–15,9y 4 groups (16–24 per group) 1. FAS, pFAS 2. Static encephalopathy, alcohol exposed but no facial phenotype of FAS (SA/AE) 1+2 with severe cognitive dysfunction 3. Neuurobehavioural disorder, alcohol exposed – mild to moderate, no facial phenotype (ND/AE) 4. healthy controls, no alcohol exposure Identified according to the 4 diagnositc digit code	4 visits during 4–6 weeks Visit 1–2: neuropsychological and sociodemographic data collection a.Quick neurological screening test II b. Wechsler Intelligence test for children III c. Wechsler Individual achievement test reading subtest + Keymath revised d. Beery Buktenica Developmental Test of Visual-Motor Integration (VMI) + Rey Complex Figure Test (RCFT) e. Delis-Kaplan-Kaplan-Executive Function System (Trail making test, tower test, color-word-interference-test, verbal fluency test) + Wisconsin morphology raw score. Raven PM and Performance IQ also high correlated.	a. Soft neurological signs b. General intellectual function c. achademic achievement (reading and math) d. Visuospatial skills, visual memory and organization e. executive function f. verbal memory g.attention h.receptive and expressive language i. adaptive behaviour j. Behavior Problems and Social Competence k. Caregiver Report of Behaviors Re-	4DDC produced 3 clinically and statistically groups Alcohol anamnese (amount) was not different! The three subgroups (ND/AE, SE/AE and FAS/PFAS) reflected a linear continuum of increasing neuropsychological impairment and physical abnormality, representing the full continuum of FASD. Behavioral and psychiatric disorders were comparably prevalent across the three FASD groups, and significantly more prevalent than among the controls. All three FASD subgroups had comparably high levels of prenatal alcohol exposure. Differences between FAS/	Controls had higher IQ than population mean	4

Anhang 4

Publikation (Autor, Jahr) Studientyp	Anzahl der Patienten Patientenmerkmale	Diagnostische Intervention/ Referenzstandard	Outcomes	Ergebnisse	Bemerkungen	Evidenzklassifikation nach Oxford
		Card Sorting test 3.ed. f. California Verbal Learning Test-Children's Version (CVLT-C) g. Integrated Visual and Auditory Continuous Performance Test (IVA CPT) h. Test of Language Development-Intermediate: Third Edition (TOLD-I:3) Sentence Combining subtest (subjects aged 8 to 10 years).Test of Language Competence-Expanded Edition Level 1.Oral Expression: R-recreating Speech Arts subtest (subjects aged 8 to 9 years).Test of Language Competence-Expanded Edition Level 2. Oral Expression: Recreating Sentences subtest (subjects aged 10 to 15.9 years.Test of Word	lated to Executive Function	PAS and Controls (% Scores < 2 SD below population mean) a. FAS/PFAS: 20 % Controls:0 % b. FAS/PFAS:15–40 % Controls:0 % c. FAS/PFAS: 5 %, 20 % Controls:0 % d. FAS/PFAS:VMI 33 %, RCFT 50–85 % Controls:VMI 0 %, RCFT 12,5 % e: FAS/PFAS: D-KFS: 0–50 %, WCST: 20 % Controls: 0 % f: FAS/PFAS: 25 %-50 % Controls:0 % g. FAS/PFAS:75 % Controls:12,5 % h. FAS/PFAS: TOWK 43 %,		

Publikation (Autor, Jahr) Studientyp	Anzahl der Patienten Patientenmerkmale	Diagnostische Intervention/ Referenzstandard	Outcomes	Ergebnisse	Bemerkungen	Evidenzklassifikation nach Oxford
Burd L. et al. **2010** Cohortstudy [19] Dakota, USA Retrospective chart review	n = 385 patients seen in a North Dakota Medical Genetics Clinic no sociodemographic data given standardized Evaluation with	Knowledge (TOWK) Conjunctions and Transition Words subtest (subjects aged 11 to 15.9 years i. Vineland Adaptive Behavior Scales (VABS) j. Child Behavior Checklist for Ages 6–18 (k. Behavior Rating Inventory of Executive Function (BRIEF), 3 criteria l. Computerized Diagnostic Interview Schedule for Children: Parent Form (C-DISC **Visit 3+4: imaging** MR-imaging **Visit 5:** results communication with caregiver Assigning an IOM Category out of chart information 1. FAS growth impairment brain dysfunction	Accuracy Groups according to IOM Sensitivity, Specificity, (False positives, False negatives, Likelihodd-Ratios	TLC-2 28 % Controls:0 % i. FAS/PFAS: 75 %, 65 % Controls:6,3 %, 6,3 % j. FAS/PFAS:20 %–65 % Controls:0 %, 6,3 % k.. FAS/PFAS:80 %, 85 %, 90 % Controls:0 %, 6,3 %, 0 % MRT results not reported in that publication 1. FAS = 152 pFAS = 151 no FAS = 87 FASDC Total Score with best accuracy 71 % FASDC total		3 b, 4?

Anhang 4

Publikation (Autor, Jahr) Studientyp	Anzahl der Patienten Patientenmerkmale	Diagnostische Intervention/ Referenzstandard	Outcomes	Ergebnisse	Bemerkungen	Evidenzklassifikation nach Oxford
	Fetal Alcohol Syndrome Diagnostic Checklist (FASDC) Diagnosed as FAS or pFAS/FAE	craniofacial features characteristic of FAS 2. Partial FAS IOM ARND or pFAS when patients did not meet IOM FAS criteria 3. NO FAS Reference Standard: IOM?!	Kappa = Measures not stated in this table) Accuracy of diagnosis without exposure (Multivariate logistic regression to estimate best-fit cut-off points for FASCD scales, Correlation between Diagnostic Instrument FASDC and IOM)	FAS pFAS no FAS Sensitivity 84,9 54,3 77,0 Specificity 82,4 83,3 90,8 1 a. FASDC no alcohol criteria FAS pFAS no FAS Sensitivity 89,3 10,4 88,5 Specificity 71,7 95,9 72,6 Classifiying subjects into FAS or NO FAS rate of agreement 58–89 % pFAS only 10–54 % agreement lowest without exposure information – data available not sufficient to produce distinctive profile ambigious classification FAs vs pFAS = 15,6 % without alcohol 19,6 % pFAs vs not FAS 9,7 % without alcohol 45,9 %		

Publikation (Autor, Jahr) Studientyp	Anzahl der Patienten Patientenmerkmale	Diagnostische Intervention/ Referenzstandard	Outcomes	Ergebnisse	Bemerkungen	Evidenzklassifikation nach Oxford
Chasnoff U. et al. 2010 [22] Case Control Study	78 foster or adopted children – 3 groups with the 4DDC Maternal alcohol use in gestation confirmed, but not amount/dosage a. n = 21 with FAS = 1. growth retardation < 3th percentile not 10th!), 2. facial dysmorphology (abnormal measurements of upper lip and philtrum Rank 4–5, and shortened palpabral fissures > 2SD below the mean 3. neurodevelopmental deficits (microcephaly < 3th percentile and/or functional deficits < 3th percentile of a test or > 2SD below the mean for more than 3 components of cognitive, executive, memory, adaptive behaviour, attentional, social skills or sensory functions	**General Intelligence** 1. Wechsler Intelligence Test for Children III 12 subtests that combine to form a Verbal IQ Score, Performance IQ score, Ful Scale IQ Score, +4 other indices Verbal Comprehension, Perceptual Organization, Freedom fro Distractibility, Processing Speed **Executive Function** 2. Behaviour Rating Inventory of Executive Function (86 behaviours of dailiy functioning that are accessible to parents) 3. Childrens Colour Trails Test 4. Wisconsin Card Sorting Test **Achievement** 5. Wide Range Achieve-	Differences in neuropsychological profile – intellectual. – executive – academic – memory, adaptive, behavioural (with X''-Test, ANOVA and MANOVA)	FAS not FAS 1 % Without alcohol 5,4 % **1. General intelligence** Multivariate analysis for 4 index socre for variance stat. sign. F= 3,63, p = 0,01 Observed power of analysis 0,981 FAS group significant lower than, pFAS (F=3,18 p = 0,019 and ARND (F=6,6 p < 0,01) pFAS and ARND not sign. Different (F=1,16, p = 0,34) **2. Memory** Overall MANOVA stat. sign. F=,38, p = 0,019 Observed power 0,880 language based memory lowest in pFAS group statistically differente only FAS vs ARND: p = 0,042 **3. executive functioning** sequencing and shiftign significant longer in the FAS grup than in pFAS and ARND Behaviour Rating without	Gruppengöße sehr stark unterschiedlich. Auswirkungen auf Effekte?! Limiation: small sample size, special group of children! Further studies with lager sample size needed	4

Publikation (Autor, Jahr) Studientyp	Anzahl der Patienten Patientenmerkmale	Diagnostische Intervention/ Referenzstandard	Outcomes	Ergebnisse	Bemerkungen	Evidenzklassifikation nach Oxford
	b. n = 10 with partial FAS = only 2.,+3. c. n = 47 with ARND = only 3. FAS children with significant less height, pFAs and ARND not significantly different. Groups similar for age, gender, racial/ethnic distribution, country of birth, adoption status, age of caregiver, rates of polydrug misuse, children welfare history	ment Test 3. edition (word reading, spelling, arithmetic) **Memory** Wide Range assessment of memory and learning screening (verbal. story, picture and design memory) **Adaptive Living Skills** Vineland adaptive behaviour scales, Interview with parents on communication, daily living and socialization **Behaviour** Child Behaviour Checklist		sign. diff. Power ok, Wisconsin Card Sortine without difference, power low. **4. academic function** No statistic difference, power 0,69 **5. adaptive functioning** differences in MANOVA p = 0,012, power of analysis 0,876 „functional communication" FAS group sign. lower than pFAS, F = 4,48 p = 0,06 ARND in between, no stat. diff. **6. Behaviour** No statistical sign. Diff., power 0,83. Authors **conclude** that FAS children are sign. Different, IQ has an impact on other tests, but can be misleading using as a covariate. High rate of attention deficit disorders in all groups		

Publikation (Autor, Jahr) Studientyp	Anzahl der Patienten Patientenmerkmale	Diagnostische Intervention/ Referenzstandard	Outcomes	Ergebnisse	Bemerkungen	Evidenzklassifikation nach Oxford
Mattson SN et al. 2010 [43] Case-Control-Study USA/Finland (2 centers of the „Collaborative Initiative on Fetal Alcohol Spectrum Disorders = CIFASD USA, San Diego and Helsinki, Finland)	Patients from the Center for Behavioural Teratology (San Diego USA) and Patients from a Research Center in Helsinki, Finland age 7–21 years (Mean age 13.0–13.7 per group n.s.) both with middle socioeconomic status levels and generally similar postnatal environments 1. Group of exposed children (> 4drinks at least once a week or > 13 drinks/week) Exposure history was confirmed via review of records or maternal report. 2. Group of nonexposed children recruited from same sites with no evidence of more than one drink per week and never more than 2 drinks on any	Standardized neuropsychological test battery, age appropriate tests in the childrens native language, limiting emphasis on verbal instructions/responses due to internationality. 547 variables from the following tests: – Edinburgh Handedness – Leiter-R – Cambridge Neuropsychological Test Automated Battery (CANTAB) – Grooved Pegboard – Virtual Water Maze,	1. **Profile Group 1 vs Group 2:** Overall accuracy of correct classification, Exposed FAS and Controls 2. **Profile Group 3 vs Group 4** Overall Accuracy and accuracy per group 3. **Comparison with IQ** 4. **Misclassified Subjects** 0. **First step:** Identification of the most discriminationg	In Discussion: Time of alcohol exposure throughput the pregnancy, and mean volume of the frontal lobes? (FAS pFAS only first trimester?) 1. **Test accuracy Group 1 vs Group 2:** Overall accuracy for Exposed/FAS and Controls/Not Fas: 92 % Accuracy Exposed/FAS: 78,8 % Accuracy controls: 95,7 % 2. **Test accuracy Group 3 vs Group 4:** Overall accuracy for Exposed Not-FAS and similar Controls: 84,7 % Accuracy Exposed/Non-FAS: 68,4 % Accuracy Controls: 95 % 3. **Comparison with IQ** FAS probands statistically sign. lower than controls	No power calculation! Limitation Sample size, Measures chosen, no validation of findings in an other group, Controls recruited retrospectively! – recall about alcohol exposure In some cases only report of the mother	3 b-4

Anhang 4

Publikation (Autor, Jahr) Studientyp	Anzahl der Patienten Patientenmerkmale	Diagnostische Intervention/ Referenzstandard	Outcomes	Ergebnisse	Bemerkungen	Evidenzklassifikation nach Oxford
	occasion during pregnancy Diagnosis of FAS only by 2 of 3 dysmorphologic criteria (short palpebral fissures, smooth philtrum, thin vermillion) and microcephaly (< 10th percentile) or growth deficiency (weight and/or height <= 10th percentile) **Categorization in 4 groups** 1. Exposed/FAS (n = 41) 2. Exposed/Non-FAS or Deferred (n = 38) 3. Control/Non-FAS (n = 46) 4. Control/Deferred or Not FAS (n = 60) Characteristics similar despite: 1. IQ Group 1 statistically lower than group 2	– Neurobehavioural Evaluation System 3 NES3- Continous Performance Test (Animals) – Visual Discrimination – Reversal Learning, – Progressive Planning Test, – Finger Localization, – Delis Kaplan Executive Function System (D-KEFS) Scored According to published test manuals, Data entered in centralized database Converted to Standard Scores according to age norms	variables, Than person-centered statistical approach by Latent Profile Analysis (LPA) = Model Based Approach, 2 class solution for profiles group1 vs group 2 and 3 vs 4 using logistical regression to evaluate the association between the groups.	(91,6. vs. 110,0 p < 0,01) IQ was not included in the initial analysis because of the goal to define a neurobehavioural profile more specific than decreased IQ. In both analyses profile significantly better than IQ alone for distinguishing Overall Accuracy IQ 75,9 % 75,6 % in the exposed group, 76,1 % in the control group. **4. Misclassified Subjects** Group 1 vs 2 = 7/2 controls Group 3 vs 4 = 16/1 control In misclassified controls any alcohol consum was denied by the parents No statistical sign. diff. Between misclassified Group members.		

Publikation (Autor, Jahr) Studientyp	Anzahl der Patienten Patientenmerkmale	Diagnostische Intervention/ Referenzstandard	Outcomes	Ergebnisse	Bemerkungen	Evidenzklassifikation nach Oxford
				0. LPA: 2 class-solution fitted best.		
				22 most discriminating variables identified covering the following functions: 1. Executive Functions (14/22) 2. Cognitive Flexibility (4/22) 3. Fine Motor (2/22) 4. Fluency (3/22) 5. Planning (1/22) 6. Sequencing (1/22) 7. Set Maintenance (1/22) 8. Spatial Learning (1/22) 9. Spatial Reasoning (4/22) 10. Sustained Attention (3/22) 11. Visual Memory (3/22) 12. Visual Motor (1/22)		
				a. **4x tests of CANTAB** (recognition memory, spatial span length, spatial working memory strategy, spatial working memory total errors)		

Anhang 4

Publikation (Autor, Jahr) Studientyp	Anzahl der Patienten Patientenmerkmale	Diagnostische Intervention/ Referenzstandard	Outcomes	Ergebnisse	Bemerkungen	Evidenzklassifikation nach Oxford
				b. 9 x tests of D-KEFS 4 Trail Making (Combined Number/Letter, Switch vs. Number, Switch vs. Visual. Switch Errors)		
				5 Verbal Fluency (Total Correct Letter, Total Correct Category, Total Correct Switch, 2nd Interval Correct, Set Loss Errors)		
				c. 1 x Morris Virtual Water Maze Test Time in Target Qudrant on Probe Trial (raw score)		
				d. 3 x Neurobehavioural Evaluation System 3 Animals Following Subtest, Number Correct, Animals Repeating Subtest, Number Correct, Animals Single Subtest, Number Correct		
				e. 2xGrooved Pegboard Test Dominant hand Completion		

Publikation (Autor, Jahr) Studientyp	Anzahl der Patienten Patientenmerkmale	Diagnostische Intervention/ Referenzstandard	Outcomes	Ergebnisse	Bemerkungen	Evidenzklassifikation nach Oxford
				Time, Non-Dominant Hand Completion time		
				f. 1 x progressive planning test maximally constrained total score		
				g. Visual Discrimination Reversal Learning Test (VDRL) Number of Reversals (raw score)		
				h. Visual Motor Integration Test (VMI) Visual Motor Integration Test Total (standard score)		
Thorne J.C. et Coggins T, 2008 [61] Retrospective Case-Control-Study	n = 32 school-aged children (8 years; 5 – 11,5) 16 with FASD, 5 with FAS or partial FAS, 16 Controls, typically developed Age-mathced, 13 also gender-matched, Not matched for IQ	Tallying Nominal Reference Errors in oral narratives (ca. 300 words) of the same wordless picture book used as a visual prompt (f. e. introducing „the „ frog instead of „a „ frog)	Diagnostic accuracy for FASD/FAS	Intercoder Agreement (out of 25 % of the material): (second coder: 10h face to face training and 40h coding practise): Kappa 0,90 [95 %CI 0,87 – 0,93]. **1. FASD vs Controls: 88 % overall accuracy'**	Exploratory, needs prospective confirmation IQ could be a confounder Controls were not neropsychologically tested	3 b

Anhang 4

Publikation (Autor, Jahr) Studientyp	Anzahl der Patienten Patientenmerkmale	Diagnostische Intervention/ Referenzstandard	Outcomes	Ergebnisse	Bemerkungen	Evidenzklassifikation nach Oxford
				2. FAS vs all others: 97 % overall accuracy cut-off 3,7 % Sensitivity 100 % Specificity 92,6 %	Comparison with a former reference error test or other variables not stated	
Vaurio L. et al. 2011 [62] Case-control-study USA, San Diego	n = 110 children aged 6 to 16 IQ matched pairs within 5 points of the Wechsler Intelligence Scale for children III as well as matched for age and SES as measured by Hollingshead a. Group 1 (n = 55) Alcohol Exposed (with FAS full or partial dysmorphological criteria) recruited by professional and self referral at least 4 drinks per occasion at least once a week or 14 drinks a week throughout pregnancy, seldom reports of the mother, records, adoption papers etc.	Application of the following tests: 1. **Receptive Language** – Peabody Picture Vocabulary Test-(PPVT-III) 2. **Expressive Language** – Boston Naming Test 3. **Verbal Fluency** – Controlled oral word association test 4. **Nonverbal Problem Solving** – Wisonsin Card Sorting Test 5. **Visual Motor Ability** – Beery Visual Motor Integration 6. **Fine Motor Ability** – Grooved Pegboard 7. **Academic Achievement**	Differences in Neuropsychological profile 1. broad neuropsychological measures 2. (items see tests) adjusted for IQ using a doubly multivariate design (multivariate analog of a matched paired t-test – the matched pair as within subject variable to maximize power, the neuropsychological outcome as dependant variable). Holm-Bonferroni for mul-	1. **Analysis of broad neuropsychological measures – a. all matched pairs** 1.-7.: marginally significant effect of group F(10,43) =2.02, p = 0,05. in univariate Follow-up Analysis sign. diff. in 4. Wisconsin Card Sorting p = 0,03) 5. Visual Motor Ability, p = 0,02 7.VRAT arithmetic p = 0,009 Alc. Exposed with poorer performance b. **because of wide IQ range – repeated analysis with 38 matched pairs** significant effect of group p = 0,029	Exminers blinded to group membership Limitations: Sample size Group selection Test selection No screening for psychopathology	3 b-4?

Publikation (Autor, Jahr) Studientyp	Anzahl der Patienten Patientenmerkmale	Diagnostische Intervention/ Referenzstandard	Outcomes	Ergebnisse	Bemerkungen	Evidenzklassifikation nach Oxford
	b= Group 2 (n = 55) controls via advertising and child-related venues, mostly reports of mothers concerning alcohol, inclusion of y 2 drinks on any occasion and up to 1 oz AA/day cave 11 % with smoking of cigarettes, 4 % Marihuana 13 (23,6 %) with IQ below the average range < 85 with no systematic reason	- Wide Range Achievement Test (VRAT) n = 3 8. Verbal Lerning Memory – California Verbal Learning Test- Childrens Version 9. Sustained visual attention – Test of Variables of Attention, Visual Subtest, 10. Child Beaviour Checklist (parent guardian reported) All Tests applied within 2–3 days in same order	tiple comparisons was used..	2. Verbal Learning and Recall 8. CVLT overall effect of group, alcohol exposed with poorer performance, but retention of verbal material no significant difference 3. Visual Sustained Attention (9.) no group differences 4. Behaviour Problems (CBCL) (10.) Overall effect of group $F(8,47) = 10,24\ p < 0,01$ Alcohol exposed group had more behaviour problems than the controls on all CBCL scales Except for somatic complaint.		

Epilepsy

| Bell SH et al., 2010, ecological study [14] | N = 425 subjects at two FASD clinics with confirmed diagnosis of FASD following the | Evaluation of prevalence of epilepsy or history of seizures in subj- | 1) Prevalence of epilepsy or/and seizures among indivi- | 1) 25 (5.9 %) with FASD had a diagnosis of epilepsy, 50 (11.8 %) had one or more | Chi-square and multivariate multinominal | 2c – |

Anhang 4

Publikation (Autor, Jahr) Studientyp	Anzahl der Patienten Patientenmerkmale	Diagnostische Intervention/ Referenzstandard	Outcomes	Ergebnisse	Bemerkungen	Evidenzklassifikation nach Oxford
	Canadian Guidelines for diagnosis. No control group. Ages of 2–49 (mean age 15.2). Age group 2–14: 51% Age group 15+: 48.5% 20% FAS or partial FAS (pFAS), 80% Alcohol related Neurodevelopmental disorder (ARND)	jects with FASD and contribution of risk factors (as prenatal alcohol exposure)	duals with FASD 2)a) Association of specific types of seizure disorders with FASD b) Association of epilepsy and/or seizures with specific subgroup of FASD (FAS, pFAS, ARND) 3) Association of history of prenatal alcohol exposure with epilepsy as an independent risk factor	seizure episodes 2) a)No difference between FASD diagnosis and risk of epilepsy or one or more seizures (p = 0.73) b) FAS group: 3 (20%9) pFAS: 10 (14.1%) ARND: 62 (18.23%) The authors describe these results as „no difference of prevalence between the groups", no p-values or CI are shown 3) History of prenatal drug exposure showed no significant results (p = 0054) for epilepsy or seizures	logistic regression were used. No control group For the results of testing the association of epilepsy and/or seizures with specific subgroup of FASD (FAS, pFAS, ARND no p-values or KI were shown. The authors describe these results as „no difference of prevalence". No separated analysis for the different age groups. There is no description about getting infor-	

138

Publikation (Autor, Jahr) Studientyp	Anzahl der Patienten Patientenmerkmale	Diagnostische Intervention/ Referenzstandard	Outcomes	Ergebnisse	Bemerkungen	Evidenzklassifikation nach Oxford
					mation with concerning maternal drinking history (self-reporting?)	
Learning, Cognition different aspects						
Simmons et al. 2010 [58]	Children aged 7–17 years Group1: n = 28 children with alcohol exposition (PAE) n = 9 with FAS, n = 19 without defined characteristics of FAS, Group 2: n = 23 non-alcohol exposed control children FSIQ and SES as variables	1. 24 trials Reaction Time: lifting forarm and Hand when stimulus light was activated 2, 48 Trials Reaction Time and Movement Task: Same as above +hitting the target keays in a designated sequence	- reaction time - reaction time and movement task (complexe movement) ANCOVA FSIQ and SES as variables Bonferroni T-Test post hoc analyses Alpha 0,05	1. Reaction time No significant differences 2. Reaction time + movement = response programming and movement time FAS significantly longer times and with more variables PAE and Controls comparable		4
Executive function/social and adaptive skills/behaviour						
Carr J et al., 2010 [20] Cohort study and ecological study,	Data were extracted from participants' clinics file of Ontario Fetal Alcohol Disorder clinic. FASD assessment was done according to Canadian guide-	Short sensory Profile (SSP) measured sensory processing ability: 38-items standardized and norm-referenced questionnaire for children between 3–18	Differences between the groups of pFAS, ARND, PEA in 1)sensory processing ability (measured by SSP) 2) adaptive beha-	1) Children with ARND scored significantly lower than children with PEA on the total score (p = 0010, taste/smell sensitivity (p = 0031) and low energy/ weak (p = 0014)	The 3 groups were compared using a multivariate analysis of variance (MANOVA). Power values of	3 b (very limited population)

Publikation (Autor, Jahr) Studientyp	Anzahl der Patienten Patientenmerkmale	Diagnostische Intervention/ Referenzstandard	Outcomes	Ergebnisse	Bemerkungen	Evidenzklassifikation nach Oxford
	lines, including an assessment for ADHD. Sample size n = 46, age between 3–14 (mean age 8): PEA group n = 15 ARND n = 16 pFAS n = 15 (no significant differences in age and guardianship)	(lower scores show more impaired sensory processing). „Definite difference" indicates performance -2.0 standard deviations below the mean. In addition to the total score, there are 7 subsections: tactile sensitivity, taste/smell sensitivity, movement sensitivity, underresponsive/seeks sensation, auditory filtering, low energy/weak, visual/auditory sensitivity. **Adaptive Behaviour System Second edition (ABAS II)** measured adaptive behaviour capability: 10 skill areas grouped into 3 broad domains: conceptional, social, practical.	viour capability (measured by ABAS II) 3) neurocognitive functioning (WPPSI-III and WISC-IV) 4) Korrelation between IQ scores and adaptive behaviour 5) Korrelation between sensory processing deficits and adaptive behaviour difficulties	2) Children with ARND scored significantly lower than children with PEA on GAC score (p = 0002). Children with pFAS did not score significantly different from the ARND or PEA group on the ABAS-II composites. 3) Children with pFAS scored significantly lower than the ARND or PEA group on Perceptual/Perfomance IQ (p = 0034). There was no significant main effect of group on Full Scale and Verbal IQ. 4) No significant correlations between any index or full scale score on IQ and any ABAS-II domains across all the diagnostic categories. 5) There was a significant positive relationship between SSP Low energy subscale with the ABAS-II GAC score (p = 0014).	0628, 0584 and 0912 were found for SSP, ABAS-II and IQ MANOVA's, respectively. Thus, implications of the the results of SSP and ABAS-II are very limited.	

Publikation (Autor, Jahr) Studientyp	Anzahl der Patienten Patientenmerkmale	Diagnostische Intervention/ Referenzstandard	Outcomes	Ergebnisse	Bemerkungen	Evidenzklassifikation nach Oxford
		Additional there is General Adaptive Composite (GAC) that reflects overall adaptive behaviour. As a measure of neurocognitive functioning **Wechsler Preschool and Primary Scale of Intelligence – 3rd ed. (WPPSI-III)** with 3 subsections (Perceptual/Perfomance IQ, Full Scale and Verbal IQ) and **Wechsler Intelligence Scale for Children – 4rd ed. (WISC-IV)** was used.				
Fagerlund A et al., 2011 [32] Case-control study and ecological study,	All children born between 1984 and 1996 and diagnosed as FASD in Helsinki were screened. The final group consisted of 73 children, FAS n = 41, PFAS=23, ARND n = 9, 60 % were girls, age range from 8–21, mean	CBCL (Child Behavior Checklist) was used to provide a syndrome profile with three broad dimensions: 1) internalizing problems such as anxiety, depressive symptoms, social withdrawl.	1) Comparison of scale scores on the CBCL between FASD group and control group 2) Association of diagnostic factors as dysmorphology	1) NC group differed significantly from FASD group on all three dimensions of the CBCL. – total problems in clinical range: 22,5 % FASD, 0 % NC (p < 00001) – internalizing problems in	– NC was not matched on social and environmental background – There was no control group assessing association of diag-	4

Anhang 4

Publikation (Autor, Jahr) Studientyp	Anzahl der Patienten Patientenmerkmale	Diagnostische Intervention/ Referenzstandard	Outcomes	Ergebnisse	Bemerkungen	Evidenzklassifikation nach Oxford
	age 13 years. 44 (60.3 %) was described with ADHD. Normal control group (NC) with N = 40, recruited through random sampling from the Finnish national population registry and were matched on age, sex, and geographical region. Maternal alcohol consumption was confirmed by review of patient records. Diagnosis of FASD was according to the revised IOM diagnostic criteria. Children were assigned a dysmorphology score (not described in more detail)	2) externalizing problems with inappropriate behaviour such as rule breaking and aggressive behaviour. 3) total behaviour problems, i. e. problems with thought and attention.	score with behaviour (measured by CBCL) was explored by a regression analyses (no control group)	clinical range: 18,3 % FASD, 2,5 % NC (p < 00001) – externalizing problems in clinical range: 14,1 % FASD, 0 % NC (p < 00001) 2) dysmorphology score after controlling for IQ, sex and age was negatively associated with internalizing problems (r_p -0357, β -0289, p < 0.05) and total problems (r_p -0229, β -0267, p < 0.05).	nostic factors as dysmorphology score with behaviour. Majority of FASD group was described with ADHD. Assessment of dysmorphology score is not described in more detail	
Nash K et al., 2011, retrospective cohort study [47]	Participants: The sample included 220 children aged 6 to 18 years, 56 with an FASD (Fetal Alcohol	10-item screening tool based on items from a standardized behavior pro-	Difference of items between 3 groups using the chi-square	1) Significant higher values in all items used Acts too young, argues a lot, can't concentrate/pay at-	Since data were collected retrospectively, certain back-	3 b

Publikation (Autor, Jahr) Studientyp	Anzahl der Patienten Patientenmerkmale	Diagnostische Intervention/ Referenzstandard	Outcomes	Ergebnisse	Bemerkungen	Evidenzklassifikation nach Oxford
	Spectrum Disorder, 4 with FAS), 50 with ADHD (Attention Deficit Hyperactivity Disorder), 60 with ODD/CD (Oppositionla Defiant/Conduct Disorder) and 53 typically developing normal control (NC) children. The FASD group was recruited from the Motherisk Follow-up Clinic, in Toronto. Inclusion: To be included in the FASD group, children had to have a documented history of prenatal exposure to alcohol and a diagnosis of ARND. Exclusion: – Children were excluded if their exposure history was unconfirmed, their primary exposure was to a substance other than alcohol (e.g. marijuana).	blems questionnaire known as the Child Behavior Checklist (CBCL). Comparison of children with FASD to children with 3 comparing groups: 1) FASD vs. NC, 2) FASD vs. ADHD, 3) FASD vs. ODD/CD FAS or ARND diagnosis is based on the Canadian diagnostic guidelines. ADHD and ODD/CD diagnosis was based on using DSM-IV-TR criteria.	test. 1) FASD vs. NC, 2) FASD vs. ADHD, 3) FASD vs. ODD/CD 4) Receiver Operating Characteristic (ROC) curve analyses were then performed for different group pairs using the sum of items most strongly differentiating each pair. Area-under-the-curve (AUC) values were used to classify cases as being FASD or NC, FASD or ADHD, and FASD or ODD/CD based on the number of endorsed items and critical cutoff values. ROC analyses	tention for long, can't sit still/resteless hyperactive, cruelty/bullying/meanness to others disobedient at home Doesn't seem to feel guilty after misbehaviour Impulsive acts without thinkung Lying/cheating Showing off clowning Steals at home Steals outside home 2) FASD also had significantly higher endorsement rates than ADHD for the following five items: – „acts young" [χ2 (1) = 5.0, p < .03], – „cruelty bullying, meanness to others" [χ2 (1) = 8.7, p < .00], – „doesn't seem to feel guilty after misbehaving" [χ2 (1) = 17.7, p < .00], – „steals at home" [χ2 (1) =	ground information was not available, particularly for the ADHD group. Finally, because the proposed screening tool is intended to be used as a screening instrument, variables important at the stage of diagnosis, such as age, family histories, and SES were not controlled for in the analyses (see demographic differences between groups).	

Anhang 4

Publikation (Autor, Jahr) Studientyp	Anzahl der Patienten Patientenmerkmale	Diagnostische Intervention/ Referenzstandard	Outcomes	Ergebnisse	Bemerkungen	Evidenzklassifikation nach Oxford
	- Any child of the comparison groups with a history of prenatal drug or alcohol exposure, defined as more than 2 drinks during pregnancy, was excluded. The NC group consisted of 53 previous control participants in other studies in our laboratory. The 4 groups were significant different with regard to SES, age, medication		lyses provide 'sensitivity and 'specificity'	17.0, $p < .00$], and – „steals outside the home" [$\chi2 (1) = 9.7, p < .00$]. 3) Children in the FASD group received a higher score than ODD/CD on only one item, namely „acts young" [$\chi2 (1) = 7.2, p < .01$]. However, children in the ODD/CD group had higher rates for being „disobedient at home" [$\chi2 (1) = 4.1, p < .05$]. 4) – Comparison of FASD and NC groups indicating the largest Area Under the Curve (AUC) was achieved with 0970 ($p < .001$); using a cutoff of 3 of 10 items, achieving sensitivity of 98 % and specificity of 42 %.	Quality of CBCL tool is not described or discussed. IQ was not assessed. Control groups were not matched for IQ For all groups, information was obtained via retrospective chart review (socioeconomic status (SES)). From each child's chart, relevant CBCL data were extracted for each case using the items from previous screener.	

Publikation (Autor, Jahr) Studientyp	Anzahl der Patienten Patientenmerkmale	Diagnostische Intervention/ Referenzstandard	Outcomes	Ergebnisse	Bemerkungen	Evidenzklassifikation nach Oxford
				– Compared with ADHD, the largest AUC was achieved with 0.78 (p < .001); using a cutoff of 2 out of 5 items, attaining sensitivity of 89 % and specificity of 54 %.		
				– Comparable ROC analysis could not be conducted between FASD and ODD/CD groups because only one item differentiated them;		
				Demographic Information: There was a significant effect of age, [F (3, 210) = 27.0, p <.01] with children in the ODD/CD being significantly older than children in the FASD, ADHD and NC groups. There was also a significant effect of SES, [F (3, 199) = 23.8, p <.00] reflected in children in the NC and ADHD having significantly higher SES than		

Publikation (Autor, Jahr) Studientyp	Anzahl der Patienten Patientenmerkmale	Diagnostische Intervention/ Referenzstandard	Outcomes	Ergebnisse	Bemerkungen	Evidenzklassifikation nach Oxford
Case-control study, Pei J et al. 2011 [54]	N = 70 (35 FASD, 35 control), aged 6–12 years, mean age 8.29 years (no significant difference between groups). Living situations were significantly different (foster care, adopted, without birth parents etc. in the FASD group) FASD diagnosis was made according to the Canadian guidelines for FASD using the 4-digit diagnostic code. Control participants were recruited form a local elementary school, matched concerning gender and age	Rey-Osterrieth Complex Figure (ROCF): a neuropsychological assessment tool that requires 1) to copy a complex geometric design with multiple details 2) then recreate the figure from memory after 3 and after 30 minutes. This test includes the Rey Complex Figure Test (RCFT) and the Developmental Scoring System for the ROCF (DSS-ROCF) as a scoring system to provide information about the degree and type of differences. RCFT involved reproducing the figure three times: Copy trial (at once), after a 3-minute Immediate Recall (IR)	Difference in: 1) „Organization" score quantifies the appreciation for the organizational goodness of complex, visually represented materials. 2) „Style" categorized the approach to information processing 3) „Accuracy" score quantifies the elements are accurately reproduced. 4) „Error" score quantifies the extent of which elements are distorted (i.e. misplaced, conflated etc.)	children in the FASD and ODD/CD groups. 1) Chi-square analyses: significant differences for the Copy trial ($p < 0001$), but not for IR or DR, with FASD group showing less favourable results. 2) Chi-square analyses: no significant differences for Copy ($p > 0126$), IR ($p > 0633$) nor DR ($p > 0943$), with FASD group showing less favourable results. 3) Chi-square analyses: significant differences on structural an incidental accuracy ($p < 0001$) for the Copy trial, but not for IR or DR, with FASD group showing less favourable results. 4) Chi-square analyses: significant differences for each of the trials. Copy trial ($p < 0001$), IR	Groups were only matched concerning gender and age, not in relation to IQ or family variables. Living situations were significant different (more children in the FASD group were in foster care, adopted, without birth parents)	4

Publikation (Autor, Jahr) Studientyp	Anzahl der Patienten Patientenmerkmale	Diagnostische Intervention/ Referenzstandard	Outcomes	Ergebnisse	Bemerkungen	Evidenz- klassi- fikation nach Oxford
		trial. after a 30-minute Delayed Recall (DR) trial. DSS-ROCF measures 4 parameters of perfor- mance: organization, style, accuracy, and error within a developmental context of age appro- priateness. Evaluations of reliability and validity for the RCFT have proved excellent.		($p < 0.05$) or DR ($p < 0.05$), with FASD group showing less favourable results.		
Memory						
Rasmussen et al. 2011 [57]	**Group 1:** 24 children with prenatal al- cohol exposure (PAE, retro- spective data), 12with FASD (2pFAS, 7 static encephalopa- thy, 3 neurobehavioural dis- order 12 without diagnosis (de- ferred) Diagnostic with 4DDC (Astley) **Group 2:** 26 controls from a local school	8 Subtests from the CANTAB (Cambridge Neuropsychological Test Automated Battery) 1. Visual (Pattern Re- cognition)and Spatial Memory Tasks 2. Executive Function and Working memory Spatial Span, Stockings of Cambridge (planning and motor skiils), Intra- Extra-Dimensional Set Shift (IED), Spatial	Statistical differ- ences in Subtests from the CANTAB, Alpha set 0,01 be- cause of numerous testing, Ancova	Children with PAE in com- parison to controls stat. sign lower in RTI (re- action time) and Spatial working memory and Rapid Visual Information Proces- sing Group differences ap- proached significance in SPAN length (executive function/working memory). Only the SPAN length dif-		4

Anhang 4

Publikation (Autor, Jahr) Studientyp	Anzahl der Patienten Patientenmerkmale	Diagnostische Intervention/ Referenzstandard	Outcomes	Ergebnisse	Bemerkungen	Evidenzklassifikation nach Oxford
	Children 6–17 years, no sign. Difference between groups	Working Memory 3. Attention Reaction Time, Rapid Visual Information Processing		ferentiated between FASD and PAE only.		

Attention

Publikation (Autor, Jahr) Studientyp	Anzahl der Patienten Patientenmerkmale	Diagnostische Intervention/ Referenzstandard	Outcomes	Ergebnisse	Bemerkungen	Evidenzklassifikation nach Oxford
Coles CD, 2001, prospective cohort study [26]	Study sample was recruited from a longitudinal cohort of 149 children (with an average age of 7.63 years) – who were of low socioeconomic status (SES) and predominantly African-American – as their caregivers. Participants were from a hospital clinic for prenatal care. 4 groups: 1) 25 alcohol-exposed children who were physically affected (i.e., had either FAS or fetal alcohol effects (FAE)) 2) 62 alcohol-exposed children who were not affected 3) control group, consisting of 35 children who had not been exposed to alcohol during	1) Focus: Selective attention to appropriate stimuli. WISC-R Coding: The child must rapidly identify and write in symbols associated with numbers 2) Shift: Appropriate flexibility in response to new information; allocation of attentional resources. Wisconsin Card Sorting Test (WCST): The child must sort cards based on one of three underlying principles: color, shape, or number	Difference in 4 attention factors: 1)Focus 2) Shift 3) Sustain 4) Encode	Children with ADHD performed less well on measures of focused and sustained attention. In contrast, children in the FAS-FAE group performed less well on measures of encoding and shifting attention.	– There is no definition or description concerning alcohol history. – Assessment of dysmorphia is not described more detailed (a checklist is mentionend, but no details are given) – No test statistics are shown, only a figure with z-scores	3 b

Publikation (Autor, Jahr) Studientyp	Anzahl der Patienten Patientenmerkmale	Diagnostische Intervention/ Referenzstandard	Outcomes	Ergebnisse	Bemerkungen	Evidenzklassifikation nach Oxford
	pregnancy but who were selected from the same low-SES population. 4) 27 ADHD-diagnosed children from the child psychiatry clinic at the same hospital where the other children were born. ADHD children were matched to the children in the study according to age, SES, and ethnic identification.	of items on card. When the sorting category is guessed, it is changed. Few ategories and perseverance on the wrong indicate lack of flexibility **3) Sustain:** Ability to maintain alert state and attention to task. – **Continuous Performance** Test (CPT) (also called Vigilance [VIG] Test): From letters rapidly displayed on a computer screen, the child must identify a predesignated signal without missing letters or responding impulsively to wrong letters (i. e., false alarms). Reaction time is also measured. **4) Encode:**				

Anhang 4

Publikation (Autor, Jahr) Studientyp	Anzahl der Patienten Patientenmerkmale	Diagnostische Intervention/ Referenzstandard	Outcomes	Ergebnisse	Bemerkungen	Evidenzklassifikation nach Oxford
		Ability to learn new material and manipulate material in working memory while processing into long-term memory. – Paired Associate(PA) Task (also called Zoo Task): Cards with animals are repeatedly paired with zoo homes of different colors. The child must recall the correct zoo when presented with the animal card – Number Recall subtest from the Kaufman Assessment Battery for Children (K-ABC) The child read a series of numbers and must repeat them accurately. – Arithmetic subtest from				

Publikation (Autor, Jahr) Studientyp	Anzahl der Patienten Patientenmerkmale	Diagnostische Intervention/ Referenzstandard	Outcomes	Ergebnisse	Bemerkungen	Evidenzklassifikation nach Oxford
Coles CD, 2002, prospective cohort study, single blinded [27]	N = 265, range 13–17 years (mean age15,1). 181 were recruited between 1980–85 from a preclinic serving a predominantly African-American, low socioeconomic population and were observed longitudinally, when their mother reported drinking during pregnancy (at least two drinks per week). Children of nondrinkers with the same SES were recruited as control group. 84 were additional recruited as control group with adolescents from special education programm. Diagnostic groups: 1) adolescents exposed/dysmorphic (DYSM)(n = 46) 2) alcohol- exposed, but not	Measures: Visual and auditory sustained attention measured with „AK" subtests from a commerciably available Continous Performance Task program. This test requires to identify a target letter „K" (either seeing or hearing) the K-ABC: The child must display basic math skills	Difference in total responses (corrects and incorrect), total correct responses (hits) and total errors (omissions, commissions, preseverations), false alarm rate, reaction time, and response sensitivity to signals 1) visual or 2) auditory presentation of stimuli between the 4 groups	Dysmorphic adolescents had significantly more responses compared with the means for the contrast and special education group (DYSM mean 37, SD 0.68; control mean 35,04, SD 0.64; EtOH mean 35.37, SD 0.51; special education mean 34,36, SD0.51 – no p-values reported, results not in tables). With the exception of total responses (Fig.1), performance of DYSM group on the visual task was significantly different (p < 0.05) from that of other groups, whereas except of the total responses performance on the auditory task was not different (p value n.s.) Visual performance:	Cognitive ability evaluated with the Wechsler Intelligence test for children differed between the dysmorphic group and the other groups. Therefore, full-scale IQ was used as a covariate in analysis of attention measures. No drop outs after 15 years? Validity of the test battery is not described	3 b

Anhang 4

Publikation (Autor, Jahr) Studientyp	Anzahl der Patienten Patientenmerkmale	Diagnostische Intervention/ Referenzstandard	Outcomes	Ergebnisse	Bemerkungen	Evidenzklassifikation nach Oxford
	dysmorphic (EtOH) (n = 82) 3) Control group: non-exposed (n = 53) 4) additional control group with adolescents from special education programm (n = 84) Cognitive ability was evaluated with the Wechsler Intelligence test for children, 3rd edition. IQ scores did not differ across the groups, except those in the dysmorphic group had significant lower cognitive scores (no discrepancy in verbal and performance IQ scores). Dysmorphia was checked on the basis of a physical examination with a „dysmorphia checklist" (Coles et al., 1985) Inclusion: adolescents exposed to alcohol/dysmorphic or alcohol- exposed, but not dysmorphic or non-exposed or			Total correct responses: p < 0003, F (3,257)=4.67 DSYM group: mean 28.96, SD 5.78 Control: mean30,9, SD 4.39 EtOH: mean 32.16, SD 4.11 Spec. education: mean 29.68, SD 6.54 Total errors: p < 0007, F (3,257)=4.07 DSYM group: mean 15.21, SD 13.37 Control: mean 9.57, SD 8.98 EtOH: mean 8.51 SD 9.33 Spec. education: mean 12.25, SD 12.39	Testers were blinded to maternal drinking history Assessment of dysmorphia is not described more detailed (a checklist is mentionend, but no details are given)	

Publikation (Autor, Jahr) Studientyp	Anzahl der Patienten Patientenmerkmale	Diagnostische Intervention/ Referenzstandard	Outcomes	Ergebnisse	Bemerkungen	Evidenzklassifikation nach Oxford
	adolescents from special education program. Exclusion: individuals with impaired physical mobility, hearing or vision or IQ < 50.					
Differential diagnosis						
Crocker et al. 2011 [28] Case-Control-Study San Diego	n = 66 children, 22 per group 7–14y 1. children with heavy prenatal alcohol exposure and ADHD = ALC (meeting DSMV-IV criteria), Mothers with at least 4 drinks per occasion/week, or 14 drinks per week during pregnancy 36,4 % with stimulant medicaments 2. Children with ADHD but without alcohol exposure 31,8 % with stimulant medicaments (ADHD) 3. control group without alcohol exposure and ADHD matched on age (within 6 months), sex and race/ethnicity	California Verbal Learning Test Childrens Version (good content, criterion and construct-related evidence of validity Results Controls as Reference Standard, Multivariate analysis	1. First: matching demographic data analyzed by Chi-Square or Standard Analysis of Variance (ANOVA) age, FSIQ, Freedom from Distractibility index Scores measured by Wechsler III and SES 2. Statistical Differences in Test Criteria Alcohol exposed vs Controls in Verbal Learning and Memory Raw Scores, Age included as variable 5	1. Demographic Information matched pairs similar on sex, handedness, race, ethnicity No significant diff. n age p = 0,09 and SES p = 0,08 FSIQ was significantly higher in the CON and ADHD group than in the ALC group p < 0,001. 2. Differences in test results stat. sign: **Group interaction significant** (p = 0,004) and also main effect of group p < 0,001. **Overall differences were apparent on all trials**, pair-wise comparison indicated		4

Publikation (Autor, Jahr) Studientyp	Anzahl der Patienten Patientenmerkmale	Diagnostische Intervention/ Referenzstandard	Outcomes	Ergebnisse	Bemerkungen	Evidenzklassifikation nach Oxford
	city All recruited as part of a longer study, via several mechanisms (CON)			the following diff. P< 0,05: CON in all trials despite 1 better as ALC ADHD sign. worse than CON on 2+3 and sign. better than ALC on 4+5 **Free Recall** after 20 min delay-CON sign better **Retention** group differences p = 0,065 ADHD worse than CON p = 0,023 ALC no sign diff to the other groups **Recognition** main effect of group significant p = 0,015 ALC more poorly than ADHD and CON p < 0,05		
Kooistra L, et al. 2011 [41]	Almost the same patients as in the following study 47 ADHD, 30 ADHD-C, 16 ADHD-PI, 30 FASD with 29 ADHD-C 39 Controls,	Continous performance tasks button press responses to target stimuli (249 trials) Go/No-Go-task button press responses	Measures of attention Response latency errors Decline in performance over time	Response latency significant effect of group F3,1=5,97 p = 0,001 ADHD-C and FASD slower and with more variables than controls Errors significant effect of group		4

Publikation (Autor, Jahr) Studientyp	Anzahl der Patienten Patientenmerkmale	Diagnostische Intervention/ Referenzstandard	Outcomes	Ergebnisse	Bemerkungen	Evidenzklassifikation nach Oxford
		to frequent stimuli and not to infrequent (210 trials)		$F_{3,105}=6,14$, p = 0,001 ADHD-C and FAS sign. More errors, but only ADHD-C significant more errors of commission 3. Performance of ADHD-C, ADHD-PI and FAS declined sign. More than that of controls over time (Go/No results not stated)		
Kooistra et al. 2011 [42]	113 children aged 7–10 years **Group 1** 47 ADHD (31 –C =combined, 16 -PI primarily inattentive) diagnosed between 5–7J 91 % on stimulants 51 % confirmed learning disability (LD) ADHD Confirmed with 3 Tests (all had to be positive): a. Summary ADHD Checklist Kaplan et al. 1997, Score 2+3 b.Conners Parents Rating Scale Revised (1997) cut-off Score > 64 on DSMV-IV Totale Scale c. Diagnostic interview for	Wechsler Intelligence Scale III for IQ: (15min) than Attention Network Test: (25 minutes) 14 practice +144 experimental trials Computer based with children making left and right responses about target stimuli with 2 fingers, congruent and incongruent flankers Tests after 24h washout	1. Demographical differences (ANCOVA) 2. Median reaction time (RT) 3. Response accuracy (MANCOVA) 4. alerting, orienting and conflict effects	Assessors blinded to groups 1. No difference for age and sex, statistically significant differences for FSIQ and SES FASD sign. lower 2. median RT ADHD-C and FAS most impaired by incongruent flankers compared to controls ($F(1,55=7,39, p = 0,02$ and $F(1,5=14,55 p < 0,01)$ ADHD-C and FAS did not differ 3. Response accuracy	ADH-PI with profile not distinguishable from controls – Number? Discriminative power limited	4

Anhang 4

Publikation (Autor, Jahr) Studientyp	Anzahl der Patienten Patientenmerkmale	Diagnostische Intervention/ Referenzstandard	Outcomes	Ergebnisse	Bemerkungen	Evidenzklassifikation nach Oxford
	children and adolescents Reich 1997/2000 also subtype assignment IQ >/= 80 **Group 2** From a FASD clinic 28 FASD Diagnosed with Fetal Alcohol Syndrome Diagnostic And Prevention Network Diagnostic Guide(DPN) 4 digit code Astley+Clarren 1999 Category G+H (H= without facial signs) Alcohol exposure 3+4 27 met criteria for ADHD and hat stimulants 13 % confirmed LD IQ >/= 80 **Group 3** 38 controls From 2 elementary school All tests negative No confirmed data for alcohol consum for group 2+3	period for ADHD stimulants		Significant effect of group not dependant from flanker type (F3,7=5,16 p = 0,02) ADHD-C had significantly lower accuracy compared to every of the other groups 4. no significant correlation in alerting, orientino or conflict effects Post hoc contrasts showed ADHD-C and FASD with higher conflicting scorse than controls		
Rasmussen et al. 2010 [56]	N = 52, 4–17 Y, with FASD (one child with FAS, 6 with	The Sensory Profile Adolescent/Adult Sen-	sensory/motor, cognition, commu-	Children with FASD and ADHD performed signifi-	Retrospective, Number of pa-	4

Publikation (Autor, Jahr) Studientyp	Anzahl der Patienten Patientenmerkmale	Diagnostische Intervention/ Referenzstandard	Outcomes	Ergebnisse	Bemerkungen	Evidenzklassifikation nach Oxford
Retrospective Case-Control Study	partial FAS, 13 with Neurobehavioral Disorder, and 32 with Static Encephalopathy according to the 4-Digit Diagnostic Code) 39 with comorbidity of ADHD	sory Profile Short Sensory Profile Bruininks-Oseretsky Test of Motor Proficiency – 2nd edition Movement Assessment Battery for Children – Second Edition (Movement ABC-2) Clinical Evaluation of Language Fundamentals – Fourth Edition (CELF-4) Clinical Evaluation of Language Fundamentals – Preschool, Second Edition (CELF-P:2) Coggins Mental State Reasoning Tasks Comprehensive Assessment of Spoken Language (CASL) Expressive Language Test (ELT) Expressive Vocabulary Test – Second Edition	nication, academic achievement, memory, executive functioning, attention, adaptive behavior	cantly worse than those without ADHD on attention but better on academic achievement. No other group differences were significant.	tients very limited	

Anhang 4

Publikation (Autor, Jahr) Studientyp	Anzahl der Patienten Patientenmerkmale	Diagnostische Intervention/ Referenzstandard	Outcomes	Ergebnisse	Bemerkungen	Evidenzklassifikation nach Oxford
		(EVT-2) Mercer Mayer Wordless Story Books (Retell, Generate, Comprehension) Oral and Written Language Scales (OWLS) Peabody Picture Vocabulary Test – Fourth Edition (PPVT-4) Preschool Language Assessment Instrument – Second Edition (PLAI-2) Renfrew Bus Story – American Edition Test of Language Competence – Expanded Edition (TLC-E) Test of Language Development – Primary, Third Edition (TOLD-P:3) Test of Narrative Language (TNL) Test of Problem Solving 2 – Adolescent (TOPS-2 A)				

Publikation (Autor, Jahr) Studientyp	Anzahl der Patienten Patientenmerkmale	Diagnostische Intervention/ Referenzstandard	Outcomes	Ergebnisse	Bemerkungen	Evidenz-klassi-fikation nach Oxford
		Test of Problem Solving – Third Edition (TOPS-3) Test of Word Knowledge (TOWK) Behavior Assessment System for Children – Second Edition (BASC-2) Conners Rating Scales – Revised (CRS-R) Continuous Performance Test (CPT) Wechsler Intelligence Scale for Children – Fourth Edition (WISC-IV) Test of Nonverbal Intelligence – Third Edition (TONI-3) Wechsler Individual Achievement Test – Second Edition (WIAT-II) or Wide Range Achievement Test – Fourth Edition (WRAT-4) Children's Auditory Verbal Learning Test (CAVLT) Rey Complex Figure Test				

Anhang 4

Publikation (Autor, Jahr) Studientyp	Anzahl der Patienten Patientenmerkmale	Diagnostische Intervention/ Referenzstandard	Outcomes	Ergebnisse	Bemerkungen	Evidenzklassifikation nach Oxford
		(also in EF) Memory subtests from the NEPSY-II NEPSY – Second Edition (NEPSY-II) Behavior Rating Inventory of Executive Function				

Tab. 3: Evidenztabelle zu Strukturellen ZNS-Auffälligkeiten

Publikation (Autor, Jahr) Studientyp	Anzahl der Patienten Patientenmerkmale	Diagnostische Intervention/ Referenzstandard	Outcomes	Ergebnisse	Bemerkungen	Evidenzklassifikation nach Oxford
Archibald S.L. et al. 2001 [3] Case-control-study	n = 14 patients with FAS (mean age 11,4y) n = 12 p. with prenatal exposure of alcohol (mean 14,8y): only few facial signs, no growth retardation FAs and PEA IQ similar n = 41 age-matched controls	MRT whole brain image 3 series 1. gradient-echo weighted T1 with cont. 1,2 mm section, 2.+3. fast spin-echos acquisitions 4 mm (2 diff. image sets)	Neuroanatomical region of interest analysis brain volume white matter, gray matter and cerebrospinal fluid was measured for each cerebral lobe and the cerebellum as well as gray matter volume of subcortical stuctures	1. Analysis done by 2 anatomists for each MRT. Interoperator reliability of total tissue volumes for independent tissue classification by 2 anatomists (using 11 brain data sets) were 0,92 for white matter, 0,95 for gray matter, 0,99 for Cerebrospinal fluid **2. Significant group differences** **FAS versus Controls** Cerebral and Cerebellar cranial vault, gray matter and white matter. (p < 0,05 each) Mediated through significant hypoplasia in the FAS group. **3. Detailed analysis:** Parietal lobe significant reduced in FAS (p < 0,05) Proportional reduction of white matter in the cere-	Analysis done by trained anatomists, blinded to participants data Diff. between PEA and Controls almost all non significant	4

Anhang 4

Publikation (Autor, Jahr) Studientyp	Anzahl der Patienten Patientenmerkmale	Diagnostische Intervention/ Referenzstandard	Outcomes	Ergebnisse	Bemerkungen	Evidenz-klassi-fikation nach Oxford
				brum p < 0,05 Parietal lobe gray and white matter reduced in FAS (p < 0,05), more than Disproportionate reduction of cadatur nucleus volume in FAS, disproportionalte sparing of hippocampal volume (relatively preserved)		
Astley et al. 2009 [10]	Group 1: N = 20 with FAS/partial FAS Group 2: N = 24 with static encephalopathy alcoholexposed Group3: N = 21 with neurobehavioural disorders, alcohol exposed Group 4: N = 16 controls with reported absence of prenatal alcohol exposure Diagnosed with 4-Digit Code Matched for age, gender, race	MRI imaging 1,5 Tesla (MR spectroscopy and functional MRI (fMRI)) and psychological and neuropsychological tests	1. size of brain/brain regions 2. correlation of FAs phenotype with brain size 3. correlation to CNS dysfunction 4. correlation with prenatal alcohol abuse	**1. size of brain/brain regions** (Only Results of FAS/partial FAS vs controls reported) Total brain volume and various regions significantly smaller in FAS/PFAS as in Controls Not significantly different in relative measures! **Mean Total brain volume** (cm³ – all measures) FAS/PFAS: 1217,8 Controls: 1370,5 p = 0,03 **Frontal lobe volume** FAS/PFAS: 346,1 Controls: 419,8 p = 0,001 **Total caudate volume**	Controls with higher IQ than mean population	4

Publikation (Autor, Jahr) Studientyp	Anzahl der Patienten Patientenmerkmale	Diagnostische Intervention/ Referenzstandard	Outcomes	Ergebnisse	Bemerkungen	Evidenz-klassi-fikation nach Oxford
				FAS/PFAS: 7,4 Controls: 9,6 ***Total putamen volume*** FAS/PFAS: 6,6 Controls: 7,6 p = 0,04 ***Total hippocampus volume*** FAS/PFAS: 5,7 Controls: 6,8 p = 0,003 **2. correlation with facial phenotype** Difference between group 1 and 2: sign smaller frontal lobe volume, mitsagittal area of cerebellar vermis, caudate volume (p < 0,05 each) **3. correlation to CNS dys-function** Significant increase of 1 or more brain regions with 2 or more SD below the Mean of the control group from Group 3 to Group 1 **4. correlation with prenatal alcohol abuse** size of various brain regions decreased significantly and		

Publikation (Autor, Jahr) Studientyp	Anzahl der Patienten Patientenmerkmale	Diagnostische Intervention/ Referenzstandard	Outcomes	Ergebnisse	Bemerkungen	Evidenzklassifikation nach Oxford
				incrementally among FASD subjects with increasing frequency, quantitiy and/or duration of reported alcohol exposure		
Björkqvist et al. 2010 [15]	Thirty-one youth (ages 8–16) with histories of heavy prenatal alcohol exposure (n = 21, 10 FAS), evaluated by 1 dysmorphologist (K.L.Jones, San Diego) and demographically-matched comparison subjects (n = 10)	MRT; structural magnetic resonance imaging, 1,5 T, T-1 weighted	Volume of gyrus cinguli, correlation to behaviour	1. Alcohol-exposed individuals had significantly smaller raw cingulate grey matter, white matter and total tissue volumes (grey and white matter together), compared to controls. 2. After adjusting for respective cranial tissue constituents, only white matter volumes remained significantly reduced, and this held regardless of whether or not the child qualified for a diagnosis of FAS. 3. A correlation between posterior cingulate grey matter volume and the WISC-III Freedom from Distractibility Index was also	Interrater correlation 0,90 +0,92	4

Publikation (Autor, Jahr) Studientyp	Anzahl der Patienten Patientenmerkmale	Diagnostische Intervention/ Referenzstandard	Outcomes	Ergebnisse	Bemerkungen	Evidenzklassifikation nach Oxford
				observed in alcohol-exposed children. These data suggest that cingulate white matter is compromised beyond global white matter hypoplasia in alcohol-exposed individuals, regardless of FAS diagnosis. The observed volumetric reductions in the cingulate gyrus may contribute to the disruptive and emotionally dysregulated behavioral profile commonly observed in this population.		
Sowell et al. 2001 + 2008 [59]	21 children, adolescents and young adults with prenatal alcohol exposure (8–22y, mean 13y). All history of heavy alcohol exposure 14/21 with FAS (mean 12,6y) 7 no facial criteria but prenatal alcohol exposure	MRI 1,5T, T1-weighted series	1. Differerence in volumes (other results of statistical parametric maps not reported) 2. Difference in cortical thickness	1. Significant group differences were observed for: Total intracranial volume $p < 0,001$ total gray matter volume $p < 0,01$ Total white matter volume $p < 0,001$ Total CSF volume $p < 0,01$ Children with prenatal al-	2001 and 2008 = same population	4

Anhang 4

165

Publikation (Autor, Jahr) Studientyp	Anzahl der Patienten Patientenmerkmale	Diagnostische Intervention/ Referenzstandard	Outcomes	Ergebnisse	Bemerkungen	Evidenzklassifikation nach Oxford
	21 controls (8–23, mean 13,3 y)			cohol exposure had in all parameters lower volumes than the controls 2. Significant group by test score interactions were found in right dorsal frontal regions for the verbal recall measure and in left occipital regions for the visuospatial measure. These results are consistent with earlier analyses from our own and other research groups, but for the first time, we show that cortical thickness is also increased in right lateral frontal regions in children with prenatal alcohol exposure. Further, the significant interactions show for the first time that brain-behavior relationships are		

Publikation (Autor, Jahr) Studientyp	Anzahl der Patienten Patientenmerkmale	Diagnostische Intervention/ Referenzstandard	Outcomes	Ergebnisse	Bemerkungen	Evidenzklassifikation nach Oxford
Yang et al. 2011 [63]	N = 69 with FASD (21 with FAS) N = 58 nonexposed controls IQ in FAS sign lower Matched fo Age (mean 13,2y) Gender, ethnicity Subjects coming from 3 sites (Cape Town, Los Angeles, San Diego)	MRI, 15,T T1-weighted series using „FreeSurfer"	1. Brain volume 2. Cortical thickness in differend brain regions (controlled for brain size)	altered as a function of heavy prenatal alcohol exposure. 1. Significantly smaller brain volume in FASD p < 0,05 2. Across and within sites FASD patients showed am overall pattern of increased cortical thickness compared with nonexposed controls (left hemisphere p = 0,028, right hemisphere p = 0,019) Cortical thickness increases were observed in the left and right inferior frontal. right middle temporal. right superior temporal in FASD (all p < 0,005).	IQ as covariate did not alter results	4

Anhang 4

Tab. 4: Evidenztabelle zu Facialen Auffälligkeiten

Publikation (Autor, Jahr) Studientyp	Anzahl der Patienten Patientenmerkmale (incl. Alter)	Diagnostische Intervention/ Referenzstandard	Outcomes	Ergebnisse	Bemerkungen	Evidenzklassifikation nach Oxford
Jones K.L, Smith D.W., Hanson J.W. 1976 [39]	N = 48 case reports of FAS up to the date of the publication whose **mothers all satsfied the criteria for alcoholism** as published 1972 by the Criteria Committee, National Council on Alcoholism	Description of principal features shared by the initial 11 children ascertained	Characteristic features of FAS	**1. prenatal and postnatal growth deficiency** prenatal growth deficiency more severe for birth length than for birth weight Postnatal Follow up up to 1 year: Average linear growth rate 65 % of normal, average rate of weight gain only 38 % Microcephaly: head circumference below 3th percentile for gestational age at birth in 10 of 11 children and after 1 year. **2. Craniofacial Signs** 11/11 Short palpebral fissures initially thought to be secondary to decreased growth of the eyes Other features commonly seen: 4/11 Epicanthal fold, 7/11 maxillary hypoplasia, 1/11 cleft palate,		4

Publikation (Autor, Jahr) Studientyp	Anzahl der Patienten Patientenmerkmale (incl. Alter)	Diagnostische Intervention/ Referenzstandard	Outcomes	Ergebnisse	Bemerkungen	Evidenz-klassifikation nach Oxford
				3/11 micrognathia. **3. Neuropsychological Characteristics** IQ from 50–83, average 63 Developmental Delay or mental deficiency 11/11 Fine motor dysfunction 9/11 **Other:** a. o. Cardiac anomalies in 8/11 patients		
Clarren et al, 1987 Case-control-Study [24]	Group 1:N = 21 7year old children with heavy prenatal alcohol exposure vs N = 21 7year old children with negligible gestational alcohol exposure (not more than 3 drinks per occasion) Groups matched for race and sex and maternal age and use of cigarettes, marijuana, valium and phenobarbital No mother used medical teratogens	Full Face and Lateral Face Photographs given to a panel of 7 expert clinicians to judge about FAS-related appearance. Morphometric analyses to identify facial differences between highly exposed and non exposed children	1. Percentage of correct Diagnosis by photos 2. Identified Differences between FAS and Non-FAS	**1.** 6 of 7 clinicians correctly identified the highly exposed children by photographs. **2.** Morphometric analysis confirmed special facial changes: short palpebral fissures relatively long and flat midface, retrusive mandibule Method to delineate more accurately the facial phenotype		4

Anhang 4

Publikation (Autor, Jahr) Studientyp	Anzahl der Patienten Patientenmerkmale (incl. Alter)	Diagnostische Intervention/ Referenzstandard	Outcomes	Ergebnisse	Bemerkungen	Evidenzklassifikation nach Oxford
Astley et Clarren, 1995 [4]	N = 194 children 2–10 years, all patients of a FAS Clinic Service in Washington, Prevalence of FAS 20 %, all evaluated in the clinic between 1/93–1/95. Randomization in 2 groups matched for age at examination, gender, race, diagnosis and date of examination	Diagnosis and evaluation of facial dysmorphology by a single dysmorphologist Group 1 = identification of patterns that discriminate best FAS –non FAS Group 2 = validation Facial Measures collected: **Eye and eyebrows** Palpebral fissure length Inner canthal distance Clown eyebrows Ptosis Epicanthal Folds Nose length **Midface** Nose Length Midface height Flat nasal bridge Hypoplastic Midface **Mouth** Smooth philtrum Thin upper lip Abnormal palate	Patterns that diagnose best FAS	**0. methods:** Discriminant analysis with step-wise variable selection (Wilks Lambda F to enter = 3,84 M F to remove = 2,71). Unstandardized canonical discriminant function coefficients were computed to derive the formula of calculation of each patients discriminant score. D-Score was ued to classify whether or not a patient was at risk for FAS. **1. Results** a. step-wise discriminant analysis selected hypoplastic midface, smooth philtrum and thin upper lip as best differentiating characteristics Sens. 100 % Spec. 89,4 % Palpebral Fissure Length and hypoplastic midface = correlation (spearman rank corr. -0,37 p < 0,000).	Reference standard cannot be independent from pattern examined, therefore not 1 b.	1 b-

Publikation (Autor, Jahr) Studientyp	Anzahl der Patienten Patientenmerkmale (incl. Alter)	Diagnostische Intervention/ Referenzstandard	Outcomes	Ergebnisse	Bemerkungen	Evidenzklassifikation nach Oxford
		Diagnosis of FAS: complrehensive evaluation by a team including pediatrician/dysmorphologist, developmental pediatrician, geneticist, clinical psychologist, educational psychologist, educational liaison, communication specialist, occupational therapist, social worker, public health nurse.		Because accurately to measure and less influencable by race, palpebral fissure length (% predicted for age) was substituted without loss of power. **D-Scores in Group 1 were plotted to identify cut-off for highest sensitivity and specificity. Cut-off was found > 1,5. = screen positive.** **Group1:** Sensitivity: 100 % (20/20 correct classified FAS) Specifity: 90,9 % (70/77 correct non FAS) **Group 2 (validation)** Sensitivity 100 % (19/19) [95 %KI97 – 100 %] Specificity 87,2 % (67/77) [95 %KI Group1+2: 85 – 93 %]		

Anhang 4

Publikation (Autor, Jahr) Studientyp	Anzahl der Patienten Patientenmerkmale (incl. Alter)	Diagnostische Intervention/ Referenzstandard	Outcomes	Ergebnisse	Bemerkungen	Evidenz-klassi-fikation nach Oxford
				Group1-2: False positive: 17/194 (12/17 with PFAE = in utero alcohol exposure, CNS dysfunction, absence of FAS facial phenotype, with or without growth retardation, 3 had other syndroms)		
Astley SJ et Clarren S. 2001 [6]	N = 952 (84 % of all patients of the clinic in Washington) with prenatal alcohol consum, mean age 6,7Y, 49 % caucasian N = 462 with Gestalt method prior to 4DDC 9,8 % FAS	Comparison of Gestalt diagnosis and 4 DDC diagnosis	% FAS diagnosed, Correlation with brain dysfunction	With 4 DDC Code 10 FAS, with Gestalt 34! Correlation to brain dysfunction and growth retardation only with 4 DDC		2 b?
Astley SJ et al., 2002, [7]. validating cohort study	Inclusion criteria: – 0 to 12 years of age at the time of enrollment, – in out-of-home placement (foster care) or – in the care of their relatives. – when a child screened positive for either FAS (with the features of the photograph) or structural/neurologic evidence of brain damage with con-	Two University of Washington students were trained to take three standardized facial photographs (frontal, ¾ view and lateral) by using a handheld, 3-megapixel, digital camera. The photographers also measured the child's head circumfer-	1) A child was screened positive for FAS if all three of the following features were present in their facial photograph: (1) palpebral fissure lengths were > 2 SD below the mean, (2) the philtrum	1) Of the first 600 children screened to date, 10 screened positive for FAS. They were 5.5 ± 3.1 years of age (range, 1.1–11.4 years), 30 % female, 40 % white, 20 % black, and 10 % native American. They all had confirmed prenatal alcohol exposure. Four of the 10 children who screened positive for FAS	20 % of the childrens' families were sent a disposable camera with a one-page pictorial instruction sheet for how to take the three standardized photographs.	1 b – (minus because a "good" reference standard according to CEBM is not available. Thus the authors used their

Publikation (Autor, Jahr) Studientyp	Anzahl der Patienten Patientenmerkmale (incl. Alter)	Diagnostische Intervention/ Referenzstandard	Outcomes	Ergebnisse	Bemerkungen	Evidenzklassifikation nach Oxford
	firmed prenatal alcohol exposure, the child was subsequently scheduled for a diagnostic evaluation at the FAS DPN clinic where he/she received a comprehensive diagnostic evaluation and treatment plan by the multidisciplinary team using the 4- Digit Diagnostic Code (Astley SJ, Clarren SK et al.) Between March of 1999 and September of 2001 screening was done. The study population comprised 600 children. They were on average 5.8 ± 4.1 SD years of age at the time they were screened, 48 % were female, 48 % were white, 32 % were black, 12 % were Native American, 15 % had documented prenatal alcohol exposure, and 32 % had	ence (occipital frontal circumference (OFC). All passports were reviewed by S.J. A. The passport was used to screen for structural or neurologic evidence of brain damage (seizures, microcephaly, abnormal brain magnetic resonance imaging/computed tomography/positron emission tomography scans, neurologic disorders) and documentation of prenatal alcohol exposure, and to generate a clinical profile. Image analysis software (Astley SJ et al.) for facial photographic assess-	was smooth (Likert rank 4 or 5 on the 5-point Lip-Philtrum Guide), and (3) the vermilion border of the upper lip was thin (Likert rank 4 or 5 on the 5-point Lip-Philtrum Guide). 2) If prenatal alcohol exposure and structural or neurologic evidence of brain damage (microcephaly, seizures of unknown origin, abnormal brain image) were present, the child was screened positive for structural or neurologic evidence of brain damage with pre-	had microcephaly and only one was significantly growth deficient (height and weight < 3rd percentile). Six had documented prenatal exposure to illicit drugs. **Diagnostic evaluations have been conducted on 7 of the 10 children** to date in this ongoing screening. **Six of the seven received a diagnosis of FAS.** 2) Fifteen (2.5 %) of the 600 children **screened positive for structural or neurologic evidence of brain damage with prenatal alcohol exposure, but did not have the FAS facial phenotype.** 3) The **prevalence of FAS in this foster care population**	to take the picture by themselves and return it by mail. For diagnostic evaluation the 4- Digit Diagnostic Code was used, published by the same authors (Astley SJ, Clarren SK et al.); no test accuracy or other details of the 4-digit code are described. Image analysis software for facial photographic assessment of the FAS facial phenotype was also released by Ast-	own developed tool as reference standard

Anhang 4

173

Publikation (Autor, Jahr) Studientyp	Anzahl der Patienten Patientenmerkmale (incl. Alter)	Diagnostische Intervention/ Referenzstandard	Outcomes	Ergebnisse	Bemerkungen	Evidenzklassifikation nach Oxford
	documented prenatal drug exposure. The FAS screening was incorporated into an already established state program, in the Foster Care Passport Program (FCPP). Public health nurse (PHN) and a health program assistant work as a team to seek out and gather all available health history information (from birth to present) for each child enrolled in the program. A shortened summary (a Health and Education „passport") is provided with health recommendations to the social worker and the foster parent to share with the child's health care provider(s). Each child's passport is updated every 6 months.	ment was used to measure the magnitude of expression of the FAS facial phenotype (short palpebral fissure lengths, smooth philtrum, and thin upper lip) from the digital images. A diagnostic evaluation at the FAS DPN clinic was done using the 4- Digit Diagnostic Code (Astley SJ, Clarren SK et al.)	natal alcohol exposure. 3) Estimated prevalence of FAS in foster care population 4) Positive and negative predictive value, sensitivity, specificity, accuracy for the FAS photographic screening tool	will be 6 of 600 or 10 of 1000 (95 % CI, 5–22 per 1000). This FAS prevalence estimates is statistically significantly greater (binomial test: P values < .001) than the FAS prevalence estimate of 1 to 3 per 1000 live births in the general population reported by the National Institute of Alcohol Abuse and Alcoholism. 4) Based on the seven screen-positive children with completed diagnostic evaluations and the 590 screen-negative children, the **positive predictive value** for the FAS photographic screening tool is 6 of 7 or 85.7 %. The **sensitivity** of the screening tool in this populationbased sample is 6 of 6 or 100 %. The **specificity** of	ley SJ et al., no test accuracy or further details provided.	

Publikation (Autor, Jahr) Studientyp	Anzahl der Patienten Patientenmerkmale (incl. Alter)	Diagnostische Intervention/ Referenzstandard	Outcomes	Ergebnisse	Bemerkungen	Evidenzklassifikation nach Oxford
				the screening tool in this population-based sample is 590 of 591 or 99.8 %. The accuracy of the tool is 596 of 597 or 99.8 %.		
Clarren et al. 2010 [25]	Normative sample of school age children (n = 1064 of 17 schools in Vancouver, British Columbia and n = 1033 of 31 schools in Winnipeg, Manitoba) to reflect the diversity of racial and national groups in Canada. The sample included students in grades 2, 4, 6, 8, and 10. Schools were selected based on racial diversity obtained from data from the 2001 Statistics Canada census. 43,1 % Male 51 % caucasian 30,3 % Asian 18,7 % other (racial/ethnical status only measured by appearance)	students were photographed in a standardized way. Photographs were analyzed using a computerized method. The palpebral fissure lengths were measured from the digital facial photographs using the FAS Facial Photographic Analysis Software.17	To analyze palpebral fissure (PF) length values and to define Canadian standard measures according to age	Analysis demonstrated that PFs do grow with age and there is a slight but meaningful difference between boys and girls in each age group. It was possible to define Canadian standards without reference to racial or ethnic origin from age 6 to age 18 with 1 and 2 standard deviations seperately for boys and girls 1. Interrater correlation reliability according to quality of photos Group A: 0,73 Group B: 0,68 Differencens in PF acording to race/ethnie not signifi-		2 b

Anhang 4

Anhang 4

Publikation (Autor, Jahr) Studientyp	Anzahl der Patienten Patientenmerkmale (incl. Alter)	Diagnostische Intervention/ Referenzstandard	Outcomes	Ergebnisse	Bemerkungen	Evidenzklassifikation nach Oxford
Astley SJ et al., 2011, [12], case-control study	Study Populations Short palpebral fissure lengths (PFL) from four existing U.S. (Washington State) study populations were used in this study. The populations were restricted to those individuals from 6.0 to 16.9 years of age to match the age range portrayed in the Canadian PFL charts. 1. Healthy School Population (1999): 90 healthy children (6.0–16.0 years of age) from a Washington State elementary school for gifted children. (47 % female, 89 % Caucasian, 1 % African American). 2. Healthy MRI Control Study Population (2003): 16 healthy children (8.3–15.8 years of age) enrolled as controls in a University of Washington FASD magnetic resonance	All PFLs were measured by one individual (Astley SJ) from digital facial photographs taken by one photographer (SJA) using the FAS Facial Photographic Analysis Software. The software computes the subject's age in years, computes the right and left PFLs in mm, and computes the PFL z-score based on which normal PFL growth charts the User selected (Caucasian5, or African American). Objectives: To assess the goodness of fit of four populations (2 groups of healthy children, children with prenatal alcohol exposure and with FAS) when plotted on	1) Graphic comparison of Canadian and Hall PFL normal growth charts 2) Goodness of fit of the healthy U. S. groups on the Canadian and Hall PFL normal growth charts. 3) Goodness of fit of the U.S. group with FASD on the Canadian and Hall PFL normal growth charts. 4) Graphic comparison of the mean PFL growth curves across published PFL normal growth charts.	cantly different (asian shorter < 1mm) 1) When the Canadian PFL charts are overlaid on the Hall PFL chart, the mean PFL growth curves for Canadian males and females fall 1.5 and 2.0 SDs below the mean, respectively on the Hall PFL growth chart. 2) The mean PFL z-scores for the school and MRI study groups were +0.17 and +0.19 respectively. Both the scatter plots and mean z-scores are reflective of a very good fit with the Canadian PFL charts. In contrast, these same children scatter, on average, 1.6 SDs below the mean PFL growth curve on the Hall PFL chart demonstrating a poor fit. (The Canadian PFL charts identify these children as	Measurement and data analysis were done by a single person (Astley SJ) using the FAS Facial Photographic Analysis Software was released by Astley SJ. Only one reviewer.	2 b (although the study is a case-control study we do not evaluate it as level 4 according to CEBM because it is a validating study

Publikation (Autor, Jahr) Studientyp	Anzahl der Patienten Patientenmerkmale (incl. Alter)	Diagnostische Intervention/ Referenzstandard	Outcomes	Ergebnisse	Bemerkungen	Evidenzklassifikation nach Oxford
	study. (50 % female, 81 % Caucasian, 6 % African American). Prenatal alcohol exposure was confirmed absent. 3. FAS Clinical Population (1993–2005): 22 individuals (6.2–13.8 years of age) with a 4-Digit Diagnosis of FAS (Diagnostic categories A and B) from the WA State FAS DPN clinical database (50 % female, 73 % Caucasian, 5 % African American). 4. Alcohol-Exposed Clinical Population (1993–2005): All 822 individuals (6.0–16.9 yrs of age) receiving a FASD diagnostic evaluation at the WA State FAS DPN (39 % female, 49 % Caucasian, 7 % African American, 10 % FAS/Partial FAS, 33 % Static cephalopathy/ Alcohol Exposed, 52 % eurodevelopmental Disorder/Alco-	the Canadian, Hall and other published PFL normal growth charts. (The Hall chart (Hall et al) is a composite of four previously published charts to measure PFL. The Canadian chart was published by Clarren et al 2010. It is a PFL chart for a racial/ethnic cross section of Canadian girls (n = 1,194) and boys (n = 903), 6–16 years of age.))	5) Assess the impact of race (specifically Caucasian versus African American) on PFL.	having normal PFLs. The Hall PFL charts identify these children as having PFLs that are, on average, 1.6 standard deviations below normal.) 3) The mean PFL z-score for the 22 children diagnosed with full FAS from the WA FAS DPN clinics was 2.4 SDs below the mean on the Canadian PFL charts and 3.9 SDs below the mean on the Hall PFL charts. These outcomes document the PFL for a child with FAS continues to fall 2 or more SDs below the mean when the Canadian PFL charts are used. The mean PFL z-score for the larger population of children with prenatal alcohol exposure was 1.1 SDs below the mean on the Canadian PFL charts and 2.6 SDs below the mean on the		

Anhang 4

Anhang 4

Publikation (Autor, Jahr) Studientyp	Anzahl der Patienten Patientenmerkmale (incl. Alter)	Diagnostische Intervention/ Referenzstandard	Outcomes	Ergebnisse	Bemerkungen	Evidenzklassifikation nach Oxford
	hol Exposed). All had confirmed prenatal alcohol exposures.			Hall PFL charts. Twenty-five percent of the children with prenatal alcohol exposure had PFLs two or more SDs below the mean on the Canadian PFL charts. Sixty-eight percent of these children had PFLs two or more SDs below the mean on the Hall PFL chart. 4) The mean PFL growth curves for the FAS Clinical Population (all FASD and the subset with FAS) was 1 and 2 SDs below the mean Canadian PFL growth curve. 5) Of the 822 patients with prenatal alcohol exposure from the FAS DPN clinic between 6.0–16.9 years of age, 400 were Caucasian and 54 were African American. These two groups did not differ significantly in mean age, gender, or FASD		

Publikation (Autor, Jahr) Studientyp	Anzahl der Patienten Patientenmerkmale (incl. Alter)	Diagnostische Intervention/ Referenzstandard	Outcomes	Ergebnisse	Bemerkungen	Evidenzklassifikation nach Oxford
				diagnostic classification. The mean PFL for the African Americans (26.5 mm, 2.0 SD) was 1.5 mm longer than the mean PFL of the Caucasians (25.0 mm, 2.1 SD) (t = 5.0, p < 0001). A 1.5 mm difference is equivalent to 1 SD on the Canadian PFL chart. In other words, if these two racial groups were plotted on the Canadian male and female PFL charts, the mean PFL z-score for the African American group (-0.1, 1.3 SD) would be 1 SD larger than the mean PFL z-score for the Caucasian group (-1.2, 1.4 SD) (t = 6.0, p < 0001).		
Fang et al., 2008, [33], exploratory cohort study	149 participants from two sites: Cape Town/South Africa and Helsinki/Finland with 86 FAS and 63 controls. Data were collected as part of an ongoing collaborative Initia-	Goal of study: To test a computational model that can automatically compute facial features from 3D scans and use this data to identify children with	1) FC sample: Sensitivity, specificity, overall accuracy 2) CC sample: Sensitivity, specificity, overall accuracy	1) FC - Sensitivity: 88.2 % - Specificity: 100 % - overall accuracy: 92.6 % Criteria: 15 features, 6 curvatures, 4 flatness, 3 aspect ratios, 2 areas	A classification system consistent with the **revised** Institute of Medicine (Hoyme et al. 2005) was used.	2 b – (a „good" reference standard according to CEBM is not avail-

Anhang 4

Anhang 4

Publikation (Autor, Jahr) Studientyp	Anzahl der Patienten Patientenmerkmale (incl. Alter)	Diagnostische Intervention/ Referenzstandard	Outcomes	Ergebnisse	Bemerkungen	Evidenzklassifikation nach Oxford
	tive on Fetal Alcohol Spectrum Disorders. Subjects were examined independently by two dysmorphologists. Exclusion: patients with recognizable craniofacial syndrome other than FAS. Inclusion: Individuals with FAS and prenatal alcohol exposure. 55 % were Finnish Caucasian (FC) and 45 % were Cape-coloured (CC), 54.4 % was female; age ranged from 2.8 to 21 years, mean age (SD) was FC 13.12 (3.5) and CC 5.09 (1.9). FC n = 82; CC n = 67	FAS. Face regions were coded with 4 features: 1. curvatures 2. flatness 3. aspect ratio 4. areas A classification system consistent with the revised Institute of Medicine was used to determine FAS diagnosis in combination with alcohol exposure (data collected through a standard questionnaire). Minolta Vivid 910 lase scanner and a novel automated facial feature analysis technique were used that compared mathematically defined surface features within selected regions of FAS and control faces.	3) Combined CC and FC	2) CC – Sensitivity: 91.7 % – Specifity: 90 % – overall accuracy: 90.9 % Criteria: 19 features, 7 curvatures, 6 flatness, 3 aspect ratios, 3 areas 3) Combined: – Sensitivity: 82.75 % – Specifity: 76.2 % – overall accuracy: 80.0 % The features for FC and CC are not specified	In this revision of IOM the CNS neurodevelopmental abnormalities were replaced by „evidence of deficient brain growth or abnormal morphogenesis, including one of following 1. Structural brain abnormalities 2. Head circumference < 10th percentile". Only limited information about this point is given (what kind of measurement was taken etc.). Thus, no neu-	able.) The authors used the **revised** diagnostic criteria of the Institute of Medicine (one of the authors (Hoyme HE) of this study is also author of the IOM paper)

Publikation (Autor, Jahr) Studientyp	Anzahl der Patienten Patientenmerkmale (incl. Alter)	Diagnostische Intervention/ Referenzstandard	Outcomes	Ergebnisse	Bemerkungen	Evidenzklassifikation nach Oxford
		To validate the diagnostic function generated from the analysis one third of the images were randomly selected and put aside.			ropsychological testing was done.	
Moore ES et al., 2007, [45], exploratory cohort study	4 Populations + control groups based on their ancestry: 1) Cape Coloured (CC), n = 103 2) Finnish Caucasian (FC), n = 99 3) African American (AA), n = 24 4) North American Caucasian (NCA), n = 50 Data were collected as part of an ongoing collaborative Initiative on Fetal Alcohol Spectrum Disorders or were recruited previously in another study. Subjects were examined by one or two dysmorphologists.	Goal of the study: To test whether computerized anthropometry can distinguish patients with FAS from controls across a wide age range and ethnically disparate study populations. Minolta Vivid 910fw laser scanner with a software package was used for merging the scans into single 3 D model of the participant's face. Identification of 16 facial criteria: **Width 7** (Minimal Fron-	1) FC sample: Sensitivity, specifity, overall accuracy 2) CC sample: Sensitivity, specifity, overall accuracy 3) AA sample 4) NAC sample	Sensitivity and Specificity as well as overall accuracy is given for the finnish caucasian population and the cape coloured population for using the 16 facial criteria (see „diagnostische Intervention") and defining maximal best distinguishing criteria for each group **1) FC** – Sensitivity:96 % – Specifity: 91 % – overall accuracy: 93 % **8 definite criteria:** (all shorter) Bitragal width Inner canthal width Outer canthal width	A classification system solely on the basis of structural features and growth deficiency consistent with the **revised** Institute of Medicine (Hoyme et al. 2005) was used. In this revision of IOM the CNS neurodevelopmental abnormalities were replaced by „evidence of deficient brain	2 b – (minus because a „good" reference standard according to CEBM is not available. The authors used the **revised** diagnostic criteria of the Institute of Medicine (one of the authors

Anhang 4

181

Anhang 4

Publikation (Autor, Jahr) Studientyp	Anzahl der Patienten Patientenmerkmale (incl. Alter)	Diagnostische Intervention/ Referenzstandard	Outcomes	Ergebnisse	Bemerkungen	Evidenzklassifikation nach Oxford
	Exclusion: patients with recognizable craniofacial syndrome other than FAS. Inclusion: Individuals with FAS and prenatal alcohol exposure. A total of 276 participants: 54 % was female; age ranged from 2.75 to 21.17 years. Only the age of the AA sample differed significantly between FAS and control group. Therefore age-adjusted regression residuals were computed.	tal. bizygomatic, bitragal. bigonial. innercanthal. outercanthal. palpebral fissure) **Depth 3** (upper, mid and lower facial) **Length 6** (Nasal. nasal bridge, philtrum, lower facial. total facial. ear) A classification system solely on the basis of structural features and growth deficiency consistent with the revised Institute of Medicine was used to dermine FAS diagnosis in combination with alcohol exposure (data collected through a standard questionnaire).		Palpebral fissure length Midfacial depth Nasal Length Nasal Bridge Length Ear Length **2) CC** – Sensitivity: 94 % – Specifity: 91 % – overall accuracy: 92 % **5 definite criteria:** (all shorter) minimal frontal width Bizygomatic width Inner canthal width Philtrum length Ear Length **3) AA:** – Sensitivity:73 % – Specifity: 85 % – overall accuracy: 79 % **2 definite criteria:** Palpebral fissure length (shorter) Philtrum length (longer) **4) NAC:** – Sensitivity:74 % – Specifity: 81 %	growth or abnormal morphogenesis, including one of following 1. Structural brain abnormalities 2. Head circumference < 10th percentile". Only limited information about this point is given (what kind of measurement was taken etc.). Thus, no neuropsychological testing was done	(Hoyme HE) of this study is also author of the IOM paper)

Publikation (Autor, Jahr) Studientyp	Anzahl der Patienten Patientenmerkmale (incl. Alter)	Diagnostische Intervention/ Referenzstandard	Outcomes	Ergebnisse	Bemerkungen	Evidenzklassifikation nach Oxford
				– overall accuracy: 77 % **2 definite criteria:** (both shorter) Inner Canthal Width Outer Canthal Width		

Tab. 5: Evidenztabelle zu Wachstumsauffälligkeiten

Publikation (Autor, Jahr) Studientyp	Anzahl der Patienten Patientenmerkmale (incl. Alter)	Diagnostische Intervention/ Referenzstandard	Outcomes	Ergebnisse	Bemerkungen	Evidenzklassifikation nach Oxford
Day N.L. et al. 2002 Cohort Study ID [30]	N = 580 Mother/Child pairs Women from an outpatient clinic May 1983 – July 1985 First interview 4th month of pregnancy > 18y, healthy, lower socioeconomic status Everage 0,6 drinks per day in 1. trimester (0–20) Assessment of 14 year old offsprings July 1998- June 2001	Interview of pregnant women a. o. use of alcohol at each trimester Assessment of children e. a. measurement of size, head circumference	Head circumference difference between children of drinking and non drinking mothers 2. Correlation between Alcohol exposure and head circumference (Controlling for Covariates: environmental variables, maternal variables, child variables, prenatal substance us other than alcohol 3. Significant predictors of head circumference (stepwise linear regression analysis)	1. Difference head circumference 6,6 mm between children of abstinent mothers or drinking 1 or more drink 2. Alcohol exposure and head circumference after controlling for significant covariates in the first trimester non drinkers: 562,74 Light drinkers (0 up to 0,2 drinks per day): 558,12 Moderate drinkers (> 0,2 and < 0,89 drinks/day): 556,95 heavy drinkers(> 0,89 drinks per day): 556,12 Average head circumference: 559 mm (503–610) No dose-related correlation in 2. and 3. trimester		2 b

Publikation (Autor, Jahr) Studientyp	Anzahl der Patienten Patientenmerkmale (incl. Alter)	Diagnostische Intervention/ Referenzstandard	Outcomes	Ergebnisse	Bemerkungen	Evidenz-klassi-fikation nach Oxford
				3. Significant predictors of head circumference ($p < 0,05$) – number of siblings – height – Gender – Race – tobacco use in first trimester		
Handmaker N. et al. 2006 [36] Cohort study	N = 209 pregnant women of n = 4460 pregnant women screened with the TWEAK and AUDIT test for alcohol use. All with risk of steady drinking (>/=1drink per day) or binge drinking (3 or more drinks per episode) at first interview (max 28 weeks of gestation) And Motivational intervention (randomly assigned to 3 different interventions) against drinking And Interview on daily drinking after pregnancy Divided in early abstainers	Comparison of intrauterine fetal growth and head circumference measured per ultrasound at 18 weeks or more up to 41,7 weeks (mean 27,1 weeks) With a Philips-ATL 3,5 or 5 Mhz by certified sonographers In 3 groups of women 1. heavy drinkers not abstaining after intervention (5 or more drinks a day n = 51)	Difference in fetal growth and head circumference (Biparietal diameter, frontooccipital diameter, BPD/OPD, Head circumference (HC) calculation from BPD/OPD, femur length, abdominal circumference (AC), indices of brain structure: transcerebellar diameter, lateral ventricular atrial diameter, diameter of	1. Comparisons between Early Abstinence and Continued Alcohol exposure no significant differences in head circumference, abdominal circumference or femure length oder BPD. Larger HC/AC Ratio with amphetamine use $p = 0,009$ **2. Comparison between early abstinence and heavy drinkers:** **ANOVA: sign. lower HC/AC-Ratio $p = 0,02$** No sign. diff. in BPD or HC alone. No alcohol effects for the		2 b

Publikation (Autor, Jahr) Studientyp	Anzahl der Patienten Patientenmerkmale (incl. Alter)	Diagnostische Intervention/ Referenzstandard	Outcomes	Ergebnisse	Bemerkungen	Evidenzklassifikation nach Oxford
	and continuing drinkers, sub-group heavy drinkers N = 56 non-drinking pregnant women	2. early abstainers after intervention Groupt 1+2 were similar for other drug use (70 % tobacco) 3. non drinkers	cisterna magnum) measured intrauterine per ultrasound Comparison with normative Data by Hadlock (1984) and By Hill (1990) ANCOVA Control of other substance use	measures of brain anatomy Lateral ventricle and cisterna magna. But significant effect for transcerebellar diameter (p = 0,008) – lower for heavy drinkers., significant decrease over time. **3. Comparison of heavy drinkers and non drinkers** HC/AC ratio significant lower p = 0,06 TDC also smaller for heavy drinkers p = 0,02 for slope? Women who abstained after the first trimester had measures not distinguishable from non drinkers **Conclusion:** singular measures do not discriminate, but ratios.		

Publikation (Autor, Jahr) Studientyp	Anzahl der Patienten Patientenmerkmale (incl. Alter)	Diagnostische Intervention/ Referenzstandard	Outcomes	Ergebnisse	Bemerkungen	Evidenzklassifikation nach Oxford
Klug et. al., 2003. [40], retrospective cohort study	The first group were subjects with a diagnosis of FAS, the second group was diagnosed with partial FAS/ARND and the third group was subjects with no FAS (who were referred for an FAS evaluation but did not receive a diagnosis of either FAS or partial FAS/ARND). They compared the growth of subjects by age, gender, and by diagnostic group. There were 1) 315 children in the sample that had weight measurements at birth and diagnosis and 2) 314 children with paired height measurements. 3) 322 children with calculated BMIs at diagnosis.	A chart review was done to assign a score or category for the criteria from the Institute of Medicine Report (IOM). During the chart review every 10th chart was independently reviewed. Where disagreement was present, the case was discussed and the categories were assigned by consensus. Each subject in the cohort was evaluated by a medical geneticist with extensive experience with FAS. A standardized examination using the Fetal Alcohol Syndrome Diagnostic Checklist (FASDC)	1) Weight measurements at birth and diagnosis 2) height measurements at birth and diagnosis. 3) calculated BMIs at diagnosis. 4) proportion of children who were below the 3rd, 5th, and 10th percentiles for growth measurements at birth and at diagnosis. Comparison between 3 groups – subjects with a diagnosis of 1)FAS, 2) partial FAS/ARND and 3) no FAS	Weight and height percentiles showed significant differences between IOM criteria ($P < 0001$), but not gender and age. Children without FAS had higher height and weight percentiles on average, though children with partial FAS had higher BMIs on average (see below). 1) Weight percentiles showed significant differences between IOM criteria (mean birth weight percentile FAS: 18 212; Partial FAS: 28 268; no FAS: 39 666; mean weight percentile at diagnosis FAS: 31 547 ; Partial FAS: 45 348; no FAS: 56 547; $P < 0001$), no difference in gender and age. 2) Height percentiles	In the section of discussion results for sensitivity and specifity, PPV, NPV and LR+/- are shown (see Anhang 7.3): Sensitivity using growth percentiles as a diagnosis of FAS. ranged from 4 to 46, specificities ranged from 71 to 100. The highest sensitivity is 46 % for birth weight 10th percentile; the highest specificity is 100 % for BMI 3rd percentile. The best PPV is 100 % for 3rd	2 b

Publikation (Autor, Jahr) Studientyp	Anzahl der Patienten Patientenmerkmale (incl. Alter)	Diagnostische Intervention/ Referenzstandard	Outcomes	Ergebnisse	Bemerkungen	Evidenzklassifikation nach Oxford
		was completed on each subject. Cases have been added to the FAS Registry continuously since 1980 (North Dakota). Paired weight and height percentiles (3rd, 5th, and 10th) from birth and diagnosis as well as BMIs at diagnosis for subjects 2 years and older were calculated.		showed significant differences between IOM criteria (mean birth height percentile FAS: 33 505; Partial FAS: 52 088; No FAS: 58 677; mean height percentile at diagnosis FAS: 30 451; Partial FAS: 36 291; No FAS: 51 196P < 0001) 3) Mean BMI differed between partial FAS (P= 0014) with higher BMI (18 315 mean percentile rank at diagnosis) than group with no FAS or FAS (mean 17 072). 4) There were significantly (p < 0.05) more children with FAS below the 5th and 10th percentiles in birth and current weight and height. Males were also more likely to be in lower birth weight percentiles. Children with FAS consis-	and 5th percentile for BMI. Limitation of the study: All subjects were only diagnosed by a single clinician. No inclusion or exclusion criteria, are described. No potential confounders are discussed. Test accuracy (validity, reliability) for the used Fetal Alcohol Syndrome Diagnostic Checklist (FASDC) is not described.	

Publikation (Autor, Jahr) Studientyp	Anzahl der Patienten Patientenmerkmale (incl. Alter)	Diagnostische Intervention/ Referenzstandard	Outcomes	Ergebnisse	Bemerkungen	Evidenzklassifikation nach Oxford
				tently have greater proportions in the lower percentiles for BMI (< 3rd %tile 22 % with FAS vs. 3 % without FAS – no level of significance shown).	No details regarding content of this test.	

Anhang 5:
Eingeschlossene Studien der systematischen Literaturrecherche

Diagnostische Kriterien des FAS

1 Abdelrahman A, Conn R (2009) Eye abnormalities in fetal alcohol syndrome. Ulster Med J 78:164–5. http://www.ncbi.nlm.nih.gov/pubmed/19 907 681.
2 Aragon AS, Coriale G, Fiorentino D, Kalberg WO, Buckley D, Gossage JP, Ceccanti M, Mitchell ER, May PA (2008) Neuropsychological characteristics of Italian children with fetal alcohol spectrum disorders. Alcohol Clin Exp Res 32:1909–19. http://www.ncbi.nlm.nih.gov/pubmed/18 715 277.
3 Archibald SL, Fennema-Notestine C, Gamst A, Riley EP, Mattson SN, Jernigan TL (2001) Brain dysmorphology in individuals with severe prenatal alcohol exposure. Dev Med Child Neurol 43:148–54. http://www.ncbi.nlm.nih.gov/pubmed/11 263 683.
4 Astley SJ, Clarren SK (1995) A fetal alcohol syndrome screening tool. Alcohol Clin Exp Res 19:1565–71. www.ncbi.nlm.nih.gov/pubmed/8 749 828.
5 Astley SJ, Clarren SK (1996) A case definition and photographic screening tool for the facial phenotype of fetal alcohol syndrome. J Pediatr 129:33–41. http://www.ncbi.nlm.nih.gov/pubmed/8 757 560.
6 Astley SJ, Clarren SK (2001) Measuring the facial phenotype of individuals with prenatal alcohol exposure: correlations with brain dysfunction. Alcohol Alcohol 36:147–59. http://www.ncbi.nlm.nih.gov/pubmed/11 259 212.
7 Astley SJ, Stachowiak J, Clarren SK, Clausen C (2002) Application of the fetal alcohol syndrome facial photographic screening tool in a foster care population. J Pediatr 141:712–7. http://www.ncbi.nlm.nih.gov/pubmed/12 410 204.
8 Astley SJ (2004) FAS Diagnostic and Prevention Network, University of Washington. Diagnostic Guide for Fetal Alcohol Spectrum Disorder: The 4-Digit Diagnostic Code 3. http://depts.washington.edu/fasdpn/pdfs/guide2004.pdf.
9 Astley SJ (2006) Comparison of the 4-digit diagnostic code and the Hoyme diagnostic guidelines for fetal alcohol spectrum disorders. Pediatrics 118:1532–45. http://www.ncbi.nlm.nih.gov/pubmed/17 015 544.
10 Astley SJ, Aylward EH, Olson HC, Kerns K, Brooks A, Coggins TE, Davies J, Dorn S, Gendler B, Jirikowic T, Kraegel P, Maravilla K, Richards T (2009) Magnetic resonance imaging outcomes from a comprehensive magnetic resonance study of children with fetal alcohol spectrum disorders. Alcohol Clin Exp Res 33:1671–89. http://www.ncbi.nlm.nih.gov/pubmed/19 572 986.
11 Astley SJ, Olson HC, Kerns K, Brooks A, Aylward EH, Coggins TE, Davies J, Dorn S, Gendler B, Jirikowic T, Kraegel P, Maravilla K, Richards T (2009) Neuropyschological and behavioral outcomes from a comprehensive magnetic resonance study of children with fetal alcohol spectrum disorders. Can J Clin Pharmacol 16:e178–e201. http://www.ncbi.nlm.nih.gov/pubmed/19 329 824.
12 Astley SJ (2011) Canadian palpebral fissure length growth charts reflect a good fit for two school and FASD clinic-based U. S. populations. J Popul Ther Clin Pharmacol 18: e231–e241. http://www.ncbi.nlm.nih.gov/pubmed/21 576 727.

13 Bearer CF, Jacobson JL, Jacobson SW, Barr D, Croxford J, Molteno CD, Viljoen DL, Marais AS, Chiodo LM, Cwik AS (2003) Validation of a new biomarker of fetal exposure to alcohol. J Pediatr 143:463–9. http://www.ncbi.nlm.nih.gov/pubmed/14 571 221.

14 Bell SH, Stade B, Reynolds JN, Rasmussen C, Andrew G, Hwang PA, Carlen PL (2010) The remarkably high prevalence of epilepsy and seizure history in fetal alcohol spectrum disorders. Alcohol Clin Exp Res 34:1084–9. http://www.ncbi.nlm.nih.gov/pubmed/20 374 205.

15 Bjorkquist OA, Fryer SL, Reiss AL, Mattson SN, Riley EP (2010) Cingulate gyrus morphology in children and adolescents with fetal alcohol spectrum disorders. Psychiatry Res 181:101–7. http://www.ncbi.nlm.nih.gov/pubmed/20 080 394.

16 BMA Board of Science (2007) Fetal alcohol spectrum disorders. A guide for healthcare professionals. Available from: http://www.bma.org.uk/images/FetalAlcoholSpec¬]trumDisorders_tcm41 – 158 035.pdf.

17 Burd L, Cox C, Poitra B, Wentz T, Ebertowski M, Martsolf JT, Kerbeshian J, Klug MG (1999) The FAS Screen: a rapid screening tool for fetal alcohol syndrome. Addict Biol 4:329–36. http://www.ncbi.nlm.nih.gov/pubmed/20 575 800.

18 Burd L, Hofer R (2008) Biomarkers for detection of prenatal alcohol exposure: a critical review of fatty acid ethyl esters in meconium. Birth Defects Res A Clin Mol Teratol 82:487–93. http://www.ncbi.nlm.nih.gov/pubmed/18 435 469.

19 Burd L, Klug MG, Li Q, Kerbeshian J, Martsolf JT (2010) Diagnosis of fetal alcohol spectrum disorders: a validity study of the fetal alcohol syndrome checklist. Alcohol 44:605–14. http://www.ncbi.nlm.nih.gov/pubmed/20 053 521.

20 Carr JL, Agnihotri S, Keightley M (2010) Sensory processing and adaptive behavior deficits of children across the fetal alcohol spectrum disorder continuum. Alcohol Clin Exp Res 34:1022–32. http://www.ncbi.nlm.nih.gov/pubmed/20 374 212.

21 Centre for Evidence Based Medicine (CEBM, 2009) Levels of Evidence. Oxford: CEBM. http://www.cebm.net/index.aspx?o=1025.

22 Chasnoff IJ, Wells AM, Telford E, Schmidt C, Messer G (2010) Neurodevelopmental functioning in children with FAS, pFAS, and ARND. J Dev Behav Pediatr 31:192–201. http://www.ncbi.nlm.nih.gov/pubmed/20 375 733.

23 Chudley AE, Conry J, Cook JL, Loock C, Rosales T, LeBlanc N (2005) Fetal alcohol spectrum disorder: Canadian guidelines for diagnosis. CMAJ 172:S1–S21. http://www.ncbi.nlm.nih.gov/pubmed/15 738 468.

24 Clarren SK, Sampson PD, Larsen J, Donnell DJ, Barr HM, Bookstein FL, Martin DC, Streissguth AP (1987) Facial effects of fetal alcohol exposure: assessment by photographs and morphometric analysis. Am J Med Genet 26:651–66. http://www.ncbi.nlm.nih.gov/pubmed/3 565 480.

25 Clarren SK, Chudley AE, Wong L, Friesen J, Brant R (2010) Normal distribution of palpebral fissure lengths in Canadian school age children. Can J Clin Pharmacol 17:e67–e78. http://www.ncbi.nlm.nih.gov/pubmed/20 147 771.

26 Coles CD (2001) Fetal alcohol exposure and attention: moving beyond ADHD. Alcohol Res Health 25:199–203. http://www.ncbi.nlm.nih.gov/pubmed/11 810 958.

27 Coles CD, Platzman KA, Lynch ME, Freides D (2002) Auditory and visual sustained attention in adolescents prenatally exposed to alcohol. Alcohol Clin Exp Res 26:263–71. http://www.ncbi.nlm.nih.gov/pubmed/11 964 567.

28 Crocker N, Vaurio L, Riley EP, Mattson SN (2011) Comparison of verbal learning and memory in children with heavy prenatal alcohol exposure or attention-deficit/hyperactivity disorder. Alcohol Clin Exp Res 35:1114–21. http://www.ncbi.nlm.nih.gov/pubmed/21 410 480.

29 D'Angiulli A, Grunau P, Maggi S, Herdman A (2006) Electroencephalographic correlates of prenatal exposure to alcohol in infants and children: a review of findings

and implications for neurocognitive development. Alcohol 40:127–33. http://www.ncbi.nlm.nih.gov/pubmed/17 307 649.
30. Day NL, Leech SL, Richardson GA, Cornelius MD, Robles N, Larkby C (2002) Prenatal alcohol exposure predicts continued deficits in offspring size at 14 years of age. Alcohol Clin Exp Res 26:1584–91. http://www.ncbi.nlm.nih.gov/pubmed/12 394 293.
31. Elliott L, Coleman K, Suebwongpat A, Norris S (2008) Fetal Alcohol Spectrum Disorders (FASD): systematic reviews of prevention, diagnosis and management. HSAC Report 1.
32. Fagerlund A, utti-Ramo I, Hoyme HE, Mattson SN, Korkman M (2011) Risk factors for behavioural problems in foetal alcohol spectrum disorders. Acta Paediatr 100:1481–8. http://www.ncbi.nlm.nih.gov/pubmed/21 575 054.
33. Fang S, McLaughlin J, Fang J, Huang J, utti-Ramo I, Fagerlund A, Jacobson SW, Robinson LK, Hoyme HE, Mattson SN, Riley E, Zhou F, Ward R, Moore ES, Foroud T (2008) Automated diagnosis of fetal alcohol syndrome using 3D facial image analysis. Orthod Craniofac Res 11:162–71. http://www.ncbi.nlm.nih.gov/pubmed/18 713 153.
34. Geuze E, Vermetten E, Bremner JD (2005) MR-based in vivo hippocampal volumetrics: 2. Findings in neuropsychiatric disorders. Mol Psychiatry 10:160–84. http://www.ncbi.nlm.nih.gov/pubmed/15 356 639.
35. Goh YI, Chudley AE, Clarren SK, Koren G, Orrbine E, Rosales T, Rosenbaum C (2008) Development of Canadian screening tools for fetal alcohol spectrum disorder. Can J Clin Pharmacol 15:e344–e366. http://www.ncbi.nlm.nih.gov/pubmed/18 840 921.
36. Handmaker NS, Rayburn WF, Meng C, Bell JB, Rayburn BB, Rappaport VJ (2006) Impact of alcohol exposure after pregnancy recognition on ultrasonographic fetal growth measures. Alcohol Clin Exp Res 30:892–8. http://www.ncbi.nlm.nih.gov/pubmed/16 634 859.
37. Hofer R, Burd L (2009) Review of published studies of kidney, liver, and gastrointestinal birth defects in fetal alcohol spectrum disorders. Birth Defects Res A Clin Mol Teratol 85:179–83. http://www.ncbi.nlm.nih.gov/pubmed/19 180 632.
38. Hoyme HE, May PA, Kalberg WO, Kodituwakku P, Gossage JP, Trujillo PM, Buckley DG, Miller JH, Aragon AS, Khaole N, Viljoen DL, Jones KL, Robinson LK (2005) A practical clinical approach to diagnosis of fetal alcohol spectrum disorders: clarification of the 1996 institute of medicine criteria. Pediatrics 115:39–47. http://www.ncbi.nlm.nih.gov/pubmed/15 629 980.
39. Jones KL, Smith DW, Hanson JW (1976) The fetal alcohol syndrome: clinical delineation. Ann N Y Acad Sci 273:130–9. http://www.ncbi.nlm.nih.gov/pubmed/1 072 341.
40. Klug MG, Burd L, Martsolf JT, Ebertowski M (2003) Body mass index in fetal alcohol syndrome. Neurotoxicol Teratol 25:689–96. http://www.ncbi.nlm.nih.gov/pubmed/14 624 968.
41. Kooistra L, Crawford S, Gibbard B, Ramage B, Kaplan BJ (2010) Differentiating attention deficits in children with fetal alcohol spectrum disorder or attention-deficit-hyperactivity disorder. Dev Med Child Neurol 52:205–11. http://www.ncbi.nlm.nih.gov/pubmed/19 549 201.
42. Kooistra L, Crawford S, Gibbard B, Kaplan BJ, Fan J (2011) Comparing Attentional Networks in fetal alcohol spectrum disorder and the inattentive and combined subtypes of attention deficit hyperactivity disorder. Dev Neuropsychol 36:566–77. http://www.ncbi.nlm.nih.gov/pubmed/21 667 361.
43. Mattson SN, Roesch SC, Fagerlund A, utti-Ramo I, Jones KL, May PA, Adnams CM, Konovalova V, Riley EP (2010) Toward a neurobehavioral profile of fetal alcohol

spectrum disorders. Alcohol Clin Exp Res 34:1640–50. http://www.ncbi.nlm.nih.gov/pubmed/20 569 243.
44. Momino W, Sanseverino MT, Schuler-Faccini L (2008) Prenatal alcohol exposure as a risk factor for dysfunctional behaviors: the role of the pediatrician. J Pediatr (Rio J) 84: S76–S79. http://www.ncbi.nlm.nih.gov/pubmed/18 758 654.
45. Moore ES, Ward RE, Wetherill LF, Rogers JL, utti-Ramo I, Fagerlund A, Jacobson SW, Robinson LK, Hoyme HE, Mattson SN, Foroud T (2007) Unique facial features distinguish fetal alcohol syndrome patients and controls in diverse ethnic populations. Alcohol Clin Exp Res 31:1707–13. http://www.ncbi.nlm.nih.gov/pubmed/17 850 644.
46. Mukherjee RA, Hollins S, Turk J (2006) Fetal alcohol spectrum disorder: an overview. J R Soc Med 99:298–302. http://www.ncbi.nlm.nih.gov/pubmed/16 738 372.
47. Nash K, Koren G, Rovet J (2011) A differential approach for examining the behavioural phenotype of fetal alcohol spectrum disorders. J Popul Ther Clin Pharmacol 18:e440–e453. http://www.ncbi.nlm.nih.gov/pubmed/21 900 707.
48. National Center on Birth Defects and Developmental Disabilities, Centers for Disease Control and Prevention, Department of Health and Human Services, National Task Force on Fetal Alcohol Syndrome and Fetal Alcohol Effect (2004) Fetal Alcohol Syndrome: Guidelines for Referral and Diagnosis. http://www.cdc.gov/ncbddd/fasd/documents/fas_guidelines_accessible.pdf.
49. National Health and Medical Research Council (NHMRC, 2009). NHMRC additional levels of evidence and grades for recommendations for develpers of guidelines. http://www.nhmrc.gov.au/_files_nhmrc/file/guidelines/developers/nhmrc_levels_grades_evidence_120 423.pdf.
50. Oxman AD, Guyatt GH (1991) Validation of an index of the quality of review articles. J Clin Epidemiol 44:1271–8. http://www.ncbi.nlm.nih.gov/pubmed/1 834 807.
51. Oxman AD, Guyatt GH, Singer J, Goldsmith CH, Hutchison BG, Milner RA, Streiner DL (1991) Agreement among reviewers of review articles. J Clin Epidemiol 44:91–8. http://www.ncbi.nlm.nih.gov/pubmed/1 824 710.
52. Peadon E, Fremantle E, Bower C, Elliott EJ (2008) International survey of diagnostic services for children with Fetal Alcohol Spectrum Disorders. BMC Pediatr 8:12. http://www.ncbi.nlm.nih.gov/pubmed/18 412 975.
53. Pei JR, Rinaldi CM, Rasmussen C, Massey V, Massey D (2008) Memory patterns of acquisition and retention of verbal and nonverbal information in children with fetal alcohol spectrum disorders. Can J Clin Pharmacol 15:e44–e56. http://www.ncbi.nlm.nih.gov/pubmed/18 192 705.
54. Pei J, Job J, Kully-Martens K, Rasmussen C (2011) Executive function and memory in children with Fetal Alcohol Spectrum Disorder. Child Neuropsychol 17:290–309. http://www.ncbi.nlm.nih.gov/pubmed/21 718 218.
55. Pei J, Denys K, Hughes J, Rasmussen C (2011) Mental health issues in fetal alcohol spectrum disorder. J Ment Health 20:438–48. http://www.ncbi.nlm.nih.gov/pubmed/21 780 939.
56. Rasmussen C, Benz J, Pei J, Andrew G, Schuller G, bele-Webster L, Alton C, Lord L (2010) The impact of an ADHD co-morbidity on the diagnosis of FASD. Can J Clin Pharmacol 17:e165–e176. http://www.ncbi.nlm.nih.gov/pubmed/20 395 649.
57. Rasmussen C, Soleimani M, Pei J (2011) Executive functioning and working memory deficits on the CANTAB among children with prenatal alcohol exposure. J Popul Ther Clin Pharmacol 18:e44–e53. http://www.ncbi.nlm.nih.gov/pubmed/21 289 378.
58. Simmons RW, Thomas JD, Levy SS, Riley EP (2010) Motor response programming and movement time in children with heavy prenatal alcohol exposure. Alcohol 44:371–8. http://www.ncbi.nlm.nih.gov/pubmed/20 598 488.

59 Sowell ER, Mattson SN, Kan E, Thompson PM, Riley EP, Toga AW (2008) Abnormal cortical thickness and brain-behavior correlation patterns in individuals with heavy prenatal alcohol exposure. Cereb Cortex 18:136–44. http://www.ncbi.nlm.nih.gov/pubmed/17 443 018.

60 Strömland K, Chen Y, Norberg T, Wennerström K and Michael G (1999) Reference values of facial features in Scandinavian children measured with a range-camera technique. Scand J Plast Reconstr Hand Surg 33:59–65. http://www.ncbi.nlm.nih.gov/pubmed/10 207 966.

61 Thorne JC, Coggins T (2008) A diagnostically promising technique for tallying nominal reference errors in the narratives of school-aged children with Foetal Alcohol Spectrum Disorders (FASD). Int J Lang Commun Disord 1–25. http://www.ncbi.nlm.nih.gov/pubmed/18 608 618.

62 Vaurio L, Riley EP, Mattson SN (2011) Neuropsychological Comparison of Children with Heavy Prenatal Alcohol Exposure and an IQ-Matched Comparison Group. J Int Neuropsychol Soc 17:463–73. http://www.ncbi.nlm.nih.gov/pubmed/21 349 236.

63 Yang Y, Roussotte F, Kan E, Sulik KK, Mattson SN, Riley EP, Jones KL, Adnams CM, May PA, O'Connor MJ, Narr KL, Sowell ER (2011) Abnormal Cortical Thickness Alterations in Fetal Alcohol Spectrum Disorders and Their Relationships with Facial Dysmorphology. Cereb Cortex. http://www.ncbi.nlm.nih.gov/pubmed/21 799 209.

Anhang 6:
Algorithmus Abklärung Fetales Alkoholsyndrom

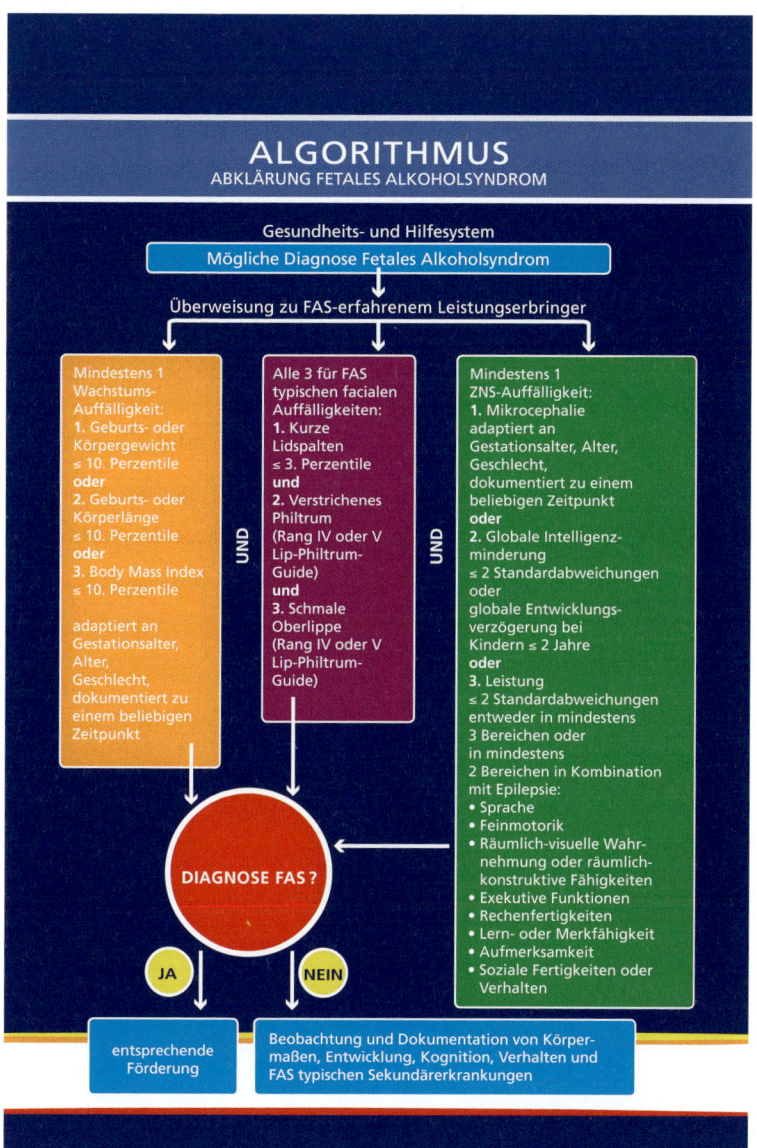

Anhang 7: Vorgeschlagene neuropsychologische Diagnostik bei Kindern und Jugendlichen mit Verdacht auf FAS

Erarbeitet von Dipl.-Psych. Penelope Thomas, Dipl.-Psych. Jessica Wagner und Dr. med. Dipl.-Psych. Mirjam N. Landgraf

Testverfahren	Abkürzung	Altersbereich
Intelligenz/kognitive Leistungsfähigkeit		
Snijders-Oomen Non-verbaler Intelligenztest	SON-R 2 ½–7 SON-R 5 ½–17	2;6–7;0 Jahre 5;6–17;0 Jahre
Wechsler Preschool and Primary Scale of Intelligence –Third Edition – Deutsche Version	WPSSI-III	3;0–7;2 Jahre
Wechsler Intelligence Scale for Children – Fourth Edition – Deutsche Version	WISC-IV	6;0–16;11 Jahre
Wechsler-Intelligenztest für Erwachsene	WIE	16;0–89;0 Jahre
Entwicklung		
Klinisch-entwicklungsneurologische Beurteilung:		
Bayley Scales of Infant Development II	BSID II	1–24 Monate
Bayley Scales of Infant and Toddler Development III	BSID III	1–24 Monate
Sprache		
Subtests „Wortschatz-Test" und „Gemeinsamkeiten finden" (WPSSI, WISC, WIE)	WPSSI-III WISC-IV WIE	3;0–7;2 Jahre 6;0–16;11 Jahre 16;0–89;0 Jahre
Skala „Sprachverständnis" (WPSSI, WISC, WIE)	WPSSI-III WISC-IV WIE	3;0–7;2 Jahre 6;0–16;11 Jahre 16;0–89;0 Jahre
Sprachentwicklungstest für zweijährige Kinder	SETK-2	2;0–2;11 Jahre
Sprachentwicklungstest für drei- bis fünfjährige Kinder	SETK 3–5	3;0–5;11 Jahre
Sprachstandserhebungstest für Fünf- bis Zehnjährige SET 5–10	SET 5–10	5;0–10;11 Jahre
Feinmotorik		
Klinisch-neurologische Beurteilung		
Movement Assessment Battery for Children	M-ABC-2	3;0–16;11 Jahre
Zürcher Neuromotorik		5;0–18;11 Jahre
Räumlich-visuelle Wahrnehmung und Räumlich-konstruktive Fähigkeiten		
Developmental Test of Visual Perception	DTVP-2	4;0–10;11 Jahre
Developmental Test of Visual Perception (Adolescent and Adult)	DTVP-A	11;0–75;0 Jahre
Abzeichentest für Kinder	ATK	7;0–12;0 Jahre

Testverfahren	Abkürzung	Altersbereich
Rey Complex Figure Test and Recognition Trial	RCFT	6;0–89 Jahre
Subtests „Mosaik-Test" (SON-R, WPSSI, WISC, WIE), „Figuren legen" (WPSSI, WISC, WIE)	SON-R WPSSI WISC WIE	2;6–7;0 Jahre **3;0–7;2 Jahre** 6;0–16;11 Jahre 16;0–89;0 Jahre
Lern- und Merkfähigkeit		
Verbaler Lern- und Merkfähigkeitstest	VLMT	6;0–79;0 Jahre
Merk- und Lernfähigkeitstest für 6- bis 16-Jährige	Basic MLT	6;0–16;11 Jahre
Skala „Arbeits-gedächtnis"(WISC)	WISC	6;0–16;11 Jahre
Exekutive Funktionen		
Testbatterie zur Aufmerksamkeitsprüfung (Untertests: GoNogo; Arbeitsgedächtnis; Flexibilität; Inkompatibilität)	TAP	6;0–90;0 Jahre
Testbatterie zur Aufmerksamkeitsprüfung für Kinder (Untertests: GoNogo; Arbeitsgedächtnis; Flexibilität; Inkompatibilität)	KITAP	6;0–10;0 Jahre
Regensburger Wortflüssigkeitstest	RWT	8;0–15;0 Jahre und ab 18;0 Jahre
Turm von London-Deutsche Version	TL-D	6;0–15;0 Jahre und ab 18;0 Jahre
Wisconsin Card Sorting Test	WCST	6;5–89;0 Jahre
Behavioral Assessment of the Dysexecutive Syndrome	BADS	16;0–87;0 Jahre
Behavioral Assessment of the Dysexecutive Syndrome (in children)	BADS-C	8;0–15;11 Jahre
Rechenfertigkeiten		
Deutscher Mathematiktest		
	DEMAT 1+	Ende der 1. Klasse bis Anfang der 2. Klasse
	DEMAT 2+	Ende der 2. Klasse bis Anfang der 3. Klasse
	DEMAT 3+	letzte 6 Wochen der 3. Klasse bis erste 6 Wochen der 4. Klasse
	DEMAT 4+	3 Wochen vor und nach Halbjahr der 4. Klasse bis 6 Wochen vor Ende der 4. Klasse
Testverfahren zur Dyskalkulie bei Kindern		
	ZAREKI-K	5;0–7,5 Jahre
	ZAREKI-R	6;6–13,5 Jahre
Aufmerksamkeit		
d2-Aufmersamkeits-Belastungstest	d2	9;0–60;0 Jahre
Testbatterie zur Aufmerksamkeitsprüfung (Untertests: Alertness, Daueraufmerksamkeit, geteilte Aufmerksamkeit)	TAP	6;0–90;0 Jahre
	KITAP	6;0–10;0 Jahre

Testverfahren	Abkürzung	Altersbereich
Testbatterie zur Aufmerksamkeitsprüfung für Kinder (Untertests: Alertness, Daueraufmerksamkeit, geteilte Aufmerksamkeit)		
Fremd- und Selbst-beurteilungsbögen zum Störungsbereich ADHS aus dem „Diagnostik-System für psychische Störungen nach ICD-10 und DSM-IV für Kinder und Jugendliche II" (DISYPS)	FBB-ADHS SBB-ADHS	3;0–17;11 Jahre 11;0–17;11 Jahre
Intelligence and Development Scales (Untertest „Aufmerksamkeit selektiv")	IDS	5;0–10;11 Jahre
Durchstreichtest vom Wechsler Intelligence Scale for Children – Fourth Edition – Deutsche Version	WISC-IV	6;0–16;11 Jahre
Soziale Fertigkeiten und Verhalten		
Elternfragebogen über das Verhalten von Kindern und Jugendlichen = Child-Behavior-Checklist	CBCL	4;0–18;0 Jahre
Youth Self Report	YSR	11;0–8;0 Jahre
Verhaltensfragebogen bei Entwicklungsstörungen	VFE-E	4;0–18;0 Jahre
Strenghts and Difficulties Questionnaire	SDQ	6;0–16;0 Jahre
Fremd- und Selbstbeurteilungsbögen zum Störungsbereich Störungen des Sozialverhaltens aus dem „Diagnostik-System für psychische Störungen nach ICD-10 und DSM-IV für Kinder und Jugendliche II" (DISYPS)	FBB-SSV SBB-SSV	4;0–17;11 Jahre 11;0–17;11 Jahre
Intelligence and Development Scales (Untertests „Emotionen erkennen", „Emotionen regulieren", „soziale Situationen verstehen", „sozial kompetent handeln")	IDS	5;0–10;11 Jahre

Güteparameter der vorgeschlagenen neuropsychologischen Testverfahren zur Diagnostik von Kindern und Jugendlichen mit Verdacht auf FAS

Intelligenz/kognitive Leistungsfähigkeit

Snijders-Oomen non-verbaler Intelligenztest 2½–7 (SON-R 2½–7)

Die Datenerhebung zur deutschen Normierung fand von Dezember 2004 bis September 2005 statt (n = 1026).

Die Reliabilität der Gesamtwerte (Handlungsskala, Denkskala, Gesamt-IQ) liegt zwischen 0,83 und 0,90.

Im Rahmen der Untersuchung der Validität wurden verschiedene Aspekte der Aussagekraft des Testverfahrens untersucht. Z. B. wurde der Einfluss verschiedener Variablen (z. B. das Bildungsniveau der Eltern auf den IQ), aber auch Übereinstimmungen und Unterschiede im Vergleich mit anderen internationalen Testverfahren analysiert. Insgesamt konnte dabei festgestellt werden, dass der SON-R „eine gute prognostische Aussagekraft" besitzt.

Snijders-Oomen non-verbaler Intelligenztest 5½–17 (SON-R 5½–17)

In dritter, korrigierter Auflage seit 2005 lieferbar, die Normen sind aus den 1990er Jahren. Die Normierung für Hörende basiert auf einer repräsentativen Stichprobe von 1350 niederländischen Kindern. Auf der Grundlage einer Stichprobe von 768 gehörlosen Kindern können Prozentränge für den Gesamtwert Gehörloser angegeben werden.

Reliabilität:

Die interne Konsistenz der einzelnen Subtests liegt über die Altersgruppen gemittelt im Bereich von $r = 0{,}71$ bis $r = 0{,}82$, die des Gesamtwertes liegt bei $r = 0{,}93$.

Validität:

Der SON-R 5½-17 korreliert zu $r = 0{,}59$ mit Indikatoren der Schulkarriere (Schultyp, Sitzenbleiben und Zeugnisnoten). Der korrelative Zusammenhang mit einem Schulfortschrittstest für Grundschüler (Cito-Test) liegt bei $r = 0{,}66$. Zusätzlich wurden zahlreiche Studien mit gehörlosen Kindern durchgeführt, die die Validität des Verfahrens bestätigen.

Wechsler Preschool and Primary Scale of Intelligence – WPSSI-III

Normierung:

- Deutschland 2009
- Alter: 3;0–7;2 Jahre

Reliabilität:

- Testhalbierung $r = 0{,}77$–$0{,}95$

Validität:

- Kriteriumsbezogen: WISC III, $r = 0{,}46$–$0{,}89$
- Klinische Validität: überprüft an Hochbegabung, leichte Intelligenzminderung, expressive Sprachstörung, motorische Entwicklungsverzögerung, ADHD

Wechsler-Intelligenztest für Kinder (WISC-IV)

Deutschsprachige Bearbeitung und Adaption des WISC-IV von David Wechsler.

Normierung:

- Deutschland 2010; 3. ergänzte Auflage
- Erhebung: von Mai 2005 bis Juni 2006 in Deutschland, Österreich, Schweiz an 2600 Kinder und Jugendlichen an über 50 Standorten
- Alter: 16;0–89;0 Jahre

Reliabilität:

- Testhalbierung (Split-half) mit Spearman-Brown-Korrektur
- r = 0,62–0,97 (durchschnittliche Reliabilität der Skalen)
- r = 0,55–0,98 (insgesamt)
- Test-Retest: wird bei deutscher Normierung nicht im Manual berichtet

Validität:

- Kriteriumsbezogen: HAWIK-III r = 0,51–0,80 bzw. r_corr = 0,59–0,89
- Konstrukt: exploratorische und konfirmatorische Faktorenanalyse; Interkorrelation Untertests und Indexwerte r = 0,21–0,92
- Klinische Validität: überprüft an Kindern mit Hochbegabung, einer leichten oder mittelgradigen Intelligenzminderung; Lernstörungen; Aufmerksamkeits-/Hyperaktivitätsstörungen; anderem sprachlichen und kulturellen Hintergrund, www.hawik-iv.uni-bremen.de

Wechsler-Intelligenztest für Erwachsene (WIE)

Deutschsprachige Bearbeitung und Adaption des WAIS-III von David Wechsler.

Normierung:

- Deutschland 2006
- Erhebung: 1999–2005 in Deutschland, Österreich, Schweiz an 1897 Probandinnen und Probanden
- Alter: 16;0–89;0 Jahre

Reliabilität:

- Testhalbierung (odd-even) mit Spearman-Brown-Korrektur
- r = 0,70–0,97 (durchschnittliche Reliabilitäten der Skalen)
- r = 0,53–0,98 (insgesamt)
- Test-Retest: nur bei WAIS-III, nicht bei deutscher Normierung
- Retest r = 0,48–0,93, für Gesamt-IQ: r = 0,96

Validität:

- Inhalt: Expertengremium und Literaturrecherche
- Konstrukt: Interkorrelation Untertests und Indexwerte r = 0,26–0,92
- Klinische Validität: überprüft an Personen, die während ihrer Schulzeit Probleme im Lesen, Schreiben, Rechnen hatten; Patienten mit Schädel-Hirn-Trauma; Patienten mit einer Major Depression; Linkshänder

Entwicklung

Bayley Scales of Infant Development-II

Normierung:

- USA 1993; BSID-II-NL, Niederlande 2002–2004
- Test auf Deutsch erhältlich
- Alter: 1–24 Monate

Reliabilität:

- Reliablitätskoeffizient α = 0,64–0,93
- Retest r = 0,77–0,91
- Interrater r = 0,75–0,96

Validität:

- Inhalt: Expertengremium
- Differenzierungsfähigkeit: Intelligenztests, Sprachentwicklungstests

Bayley Scales of Infant and Toddlers Development-III

Normierung:

- USA 2004
- Test auf Deutsch erhältlich
- Alter: 1–24 Monate

Reliabilität:

- Interne Kosistenz: Split-Half r = 0,76–0,94
- Retest r = 0,71–0,92
- Interrater r = 0,59–0,86

Validität:

- Differenzierungsfähigkeit: andere Tests
- klinisch: Down-Syndrom, Entwicklungsstörung, Cerebralparese, perinatale Asphyxie, pränatale Alkoholexposition, SGA, Frühgeborene, motorische und physische Behinderung, rezeptive und expressive Sprachstörung

Teilbereiche funktioneller ZNS-Auffälligkeiten

1 Sprache

Sprachentwicklungstest für zweijährige Kinder SETK-2

Normierung:

- Deutschland 2000
- Alter: 2;0–2;11 Jahre

Reliabilität:

- Interne Konsistenz α = 0,56–0,95

Validität:

- Konstrukt: Interkorrelation Untertests r = 0,55–0,82
- Konvergente Validität: Elternberichte r = 0,77–0,84
- Differenzierungsfähigkeit getestet signifikant gg. Hörprobleme, Frühgeborene
- Prognostische Validität: späte Wortlerner r = 0,6–0,7

Sprachentwicklungstest für drei- bis fünfjährige Kinder SETK 3–5

Normierung:

- Deutschland 2001
- Alter: 3;0–5;11 Jahre

Reliabilität:

- Interne Konsistenz α = 0,62–0,89

Validität:

- Konstrukt: Interkorrelation Untertests r = 0,22–0,66
- Differenzierungsfähigkeit getestet signifikant gg. dysphasisch sprachgestörte Kindern, Frühgeborene, Late Talker

Sprachstandserhebungstest für Fünf- bis Zehnjährige SET 5–10

Normierung:

- Deutschland 2009
- Alter: 5;0–10;11 Jahre

Reliabilität:

- Interne Konsistenz α = 0,61–0,91

Validität:

- im Manual nicht evaluiert.

2 Feinmotorik

Movement Assessment Battery for Children M-ABC-2

(Handgeschicklichkeit, Ballfertigkeit, Balance)

Normierung:

- Originalnormen 2005–2006 Großbritannien und Nordirland
- Deutsche Vergleichsstudie 2007/2008 – Normen für Deutschland bestätigt
- Alter: 3;0–6;11, 7;0–10;11 und 11;0–16;11 Jahre (3 Testbatterien)

Reliabilität:

- Retest r = 0,62–0,92
- Interrater r = 0,92–1,0

Validität:

- Inhaltsvalidität: Skalen korreliert mit Gesamtwert r = 0,65–0,76 und Expertengremium
- Kriteriumsvalidität: Korrelation mit Mann-Zeichen-Test r = 0,66
- Klinische Validierungsstudien (Umschriebene Entwicklungsstörung motorischer Funktionen, Sprachstörungen, ADHS, Autistische Störungen, Lernstörungen, Intelligenzminderung)

Zürcher Neuromotorik

(Repetitive Bewegungen; Alternierende Bewegungen; Sequentielle Bewegungen; Adaptive Leistungen; Gleichgewicht; Haltung)

Normierung:

- Schweiz 1997
- Alter: 5;0–18;11 Jahre

Reliabilität:

- Zeitmessung:
  – Intra-Rater: r = 0,56–1,0
  – Inter-Rater: r = 0,32–0,99
  – Test-Retest: r = 0,38–0,89
- Mitbewegungen:
  – Intra-Rater: r = 0,53–0,90
  – Inter-Rater: r = 0,44–0,82
  – Test-Retest: r = 0,20–0,61

- Indizes:
  - Intra-Rater: r = 0,73–1,0
  - Inter-Rater: r = 0,62–0,98
  - Test-Retest: r = 0,40–0,91

Validität:

- Klinische Validität: motorische Ungeschicklichkeit, die pädagogischer oder medizinischer Intervention bedurfte, Frühgeborene, angeborener Herzfehler, Z. n. perinataler Asphyxie, spezifische Spracherwerbsstörung.

Sensitivität: 93 %
Spezifität: 93 %

3 Räumlich-visuelle Wahrnehmung und Räumlich-konstruktive Fähigkeiten

Developmental Test of Visual Perception DTVP-2

Normierung:

- USA 1992
- Alter: 4;0–10;11 Jahre
- Test nur auf Englisch, jedoch Beurteilung nicht sprachgebundener Leistungen

Reliabilität:

- Content Sampling α = 0,83–0,95
- Interne Konsistenz α = 0,77–0,96
- Retest r = 0,71–0,86
- Interrater r = 0,93–0,99

Validität:

- Kriteriumsbezogen: MVPT r = 0,65
- Inhalt und Konstrukt ebenfalls evaluiert

Developmental Test of Visual Perception DTVP-A (Adolescent and Adult)

Normierung:

- USA 2002
- Alter: 11;0–75;0 Jahre
- Test nur auf Englisch, jedoch Beurteilung nicht sprachgebundener Leistungen (Erhebung 1999–2000 in den USA an 1664 Personen in 19 Staaten)

Reliabilität:

- Content Sampling (subtests) α = 0,77–0,89
- Content Sampling (indexes) α = 0,85–0,93
- Retest r = 0,70–0,84
- Interrater r = 0,94–0,99

Validität:

- Kriteriumsbezogen: RCFT (DTVP-A Indexes; immediate recall) r = 0,48–0,78
- Kriteriumsbezogen: RCFT (DTVP-A Indexes; delayed recall) r = 0,52–0,64
- Kriteriumsbezogen: DAP: IQ (Draw a person) und DTVP Index: r = 0,36–0,42
- Kriteriumsbezogen: CTMT (Comprehensive Trail Making Test) und DTVP-Index: r = 0,40–0,76
- Inhalt und Konstrukt ebenfalls evaluiert; laut Autoren ist Inhaltsvalidität (Testmanual S. 66) und Konstruktvalidität (konfirmatorische Faktorenanalyse; Testmanual S. 74) gegeben.

Abzeichentest für Kinder (ATK)

(Neubearbeitung in Anlehnung an den Itempool des Gailinger Abzeichentest mit Markierungshilfen, GAT)

Normierung:

- Deutschland 2004 (Erhebung an 350 gesunden Kindern)
- Alter: 7;0–12;0 Jahre

Reliabilität: bisher keine Angaben dazu.

Validität: Konstrukt:

- Klinik: neurologische Stichprobe von Kindern mit gesicherter räumlich-konstruktiver Störung und neurologische Stichprobe von Kindern ohne räumlich-konstruktive Störung.
- Korrelation des GAT und Mosaiktest (MT) aus HAWIK: r = 0,50
- Cut-off-Wert (ATK) und Wertpunkt von ≤ 4 (MT): Übereinstimmung von 87,5 %; die Autoren gehen daher von einer guten klinischen Validität des ATK aus (S. 30).

Rey Complex Figure Test and Recognition Trial RCFT

(visuell-räumliches Gedächtnis und visuell-räumliche Konstrukt-Fähigkeiten)

Normierung:

- USA 1993
- Alter: 6;0–89;0 Jahre

- Test nur auf Englisch, jedoch Beurteilung nicht sprachgebundener Leistungen

Reliabilität:

- Interrater r = 0,93–0,99
- Retest r = 0,76–0,89

Validität:

- Konstrukt: Klinik: Gehirnschäden
- Korrelation mit Subtests anderer neuropsycholog. Testverfahren
- Diskrimination Gesund/psychiatrisch krank/Gehirnschaden
  - Copy: richtig positiv 57,8 %
  - Recall: richtig positiv 61,1 %
  - Recall and Recognition richtig positiv 77,8 %

4 Exekutive Funktionen

Testbatterie zur Aufmerksamkeitsprüfung (TAP)

Version 2.3 (Version 2012)

Normierung:

- Deutschland 2007
- Erhebung: Normierungsdaten aus unterschiedlichen Studien, aus denen jeweils unterschiedliche Teilmengen von Tests verwendet wurden
- Tests sind nicht in gleichem Umfang für Erwachsene und Jugendliche normiert
- Alter: 6;0– 90;0 Jahre (abhängig vom jeweiligen Untertest)

Reliabilität:

- Testhalbierung (Odd-Even-Reliabilität): r = 0,219–0,997 (insgesamt für alle Tests; Kinder- und Jugendliche: 6–19 Jahre);
- Insgesamt: die Reliabilitäten der Reaktionszeitmediane liegen überwiegend über 0,90, daher zufriedenstellend bis sehr gut; die Reliabilitäten der Fehlermaße sind hingegen häufig unzureichend;
- Test-Retest: siehe vorläufige Ergebnisse für Erwachsene (Test-Manual: S. 99–100); Es liegt eine Studie von Földényi et al. (2000) zur Reliabilität und Retest-Stabilität bei 95 Deutschschweizer Schulkindern vor (7–10 Jahre): r_tt = 0,84; insgesamt mittlere bis hohe Reliabilitäten mit Ausnahme des Untertests: Geteilte Aufmerksamkeit: r_tt = 0,32; insgesamt: deutlich bessere Reliabilitäten bei Reaktionszeitmedianen im Vergleich zu Kriterien der Leistungsgüte (Auslassungen, Fehler).

Validität:

- Konstrukt: Studien zur faktoriellen Validität liegen vor.
- Klinische Validität: Studien mit neurologischen Patienten, psychiatrischen Patienten, pharmakologische Studien, funktionelle Bildgebungsstudien, Studien mit Kindern und Studien mit älteren Probanden; Studien mit Kindern:
  - Földényi et al. (2000): klinische Validierungsstudie an Kindern mit ADHS: 90 % der Kinder konnten korrekt der ADHS-Gruppe oder Kontrollgruppe zugeordnet werden anhand Reaktionszeit-Schwankungen im Go/Nogo, Fehleranzahl bei Flexibilität (Wechsel: nonverbal) und Testalter; Kriteriumsvalidität: Korrelation TAP und Eltern-/Lehrerurteile (standardisierte Fragebögen): signifikante Korrelation Go/Nogo, Inkompatibilität, geteilte Aufmerksamkeit, Flexibilität
  - Koschak et al. (2003): ADHS-Kontrollgruppe
  - Tucha et al. (2005): ADHS-Gesunde Kinder
  - Heubrock et al. (2001): Inanspruchnahme neuropsychologischer Ambulanz
  - Kunert et al. (1996): faktorielle Validität

Testbatterie zur Aufmerksamkeitsprüfung für Kinder (KITAP)

Normierung:

- Deutschland 2002
- Erhebung: Normierungsdaten aus unterschiedlichen Studien, aus denen jeweils unterschiedliche Teilmengen von Tests verwendet wurden aus Deutschland, Frankreich, Belgien, Italien, Schweiz, Österreich
- Alter: 6;0–10;0 Jahre

Reliabilität:

- Testhalbierung (Split-Half-Reliabilität):
- r = 0,64–0,97 (insgesamt für alle Tests; Kinder: 6–7 Jahre)
- r = 0,63–0,96 (insgesamt für alle Tests; Kinder: 8–10 Jahre)
- Insgesamt: die Reliabilitäten der Reaktionszeitmediane deutlich besser, z. T. sehr gut; die Reliabilitäten der Fehlermaße sind hingegen häufig im unteren Bereich, aufgrund insgesamt eher geringer Auslassungen als Artefakte zu betrachten.

Validität:

- Konstrukt: Studien zur faktoriellen Validität liegen vor.
- Klinische Validität: Studien bei Kindern mit ADHS und nach Hirnschädigung

Regensburger Wortflüssigkeitstest (RWT)

Die Normen stammen aus dem Jahr 2000 (n (Kinder) = 184).

Reliabilität:

Keine Angaben zur internen Konsistenz. Retest-Reliabilitätskoeffizienten zwischen 0,72 und 0,89 (N = 80). Interrater-Reliabilität = 0,99.

Validität:

Die Autoren verweisen auf die umfangreiche Literatur zu diesem gut eingeführten Verfahren. Für eine Unterstichprobe (N = 94) wurden außerdem Korrelationen mit Leistungen in IQ- und anderen neuropsychologischen Tests berechnet. Am höchsten korrelieren die Ergebnisse mit einem Test zur figuralen Flüssigkeit (5-Punkte-Test, Regard 1982; Korrelation mit S-Wörtern r =.512). Bezüglich der klinischen Validität verweisen die Autoren auf die Sensibilität dieses etablierten Verfahrens für verschiedene klinische Gruppen und auf die Ergebnisse in denen von ihnen erhobenen Patientengruppen.

Turm von London – Deutsche Version (TL-D; Tucha und Lange 2004)

Der Test in der deutschen Version beinhaltet insgesamt 20 Aufgaben, die komplexe Planungsprozesse erfordern. Der Testaufbau besteht aus 3 verschiedenfarbigen Kugeln, die auf 3 nebeneinander angeordneten Stäben von unterschiedlicher Länge angeordnet sind. Auf den Stäben ist entweder Platz für eine, zwei oder drei Kugeln. Der Proband soll dabei von einem Ausgangszustand zu einem Zielzustand kommen, d. h. er soll in minimalen Zügen die Kugeln so verändern, dass es mit dem Zielbild übereinstimmt. Pro Zug darf jedoch nur eine Kugel verwendet werden. Der Schwierigkeitsgrad nimmt bei den 20 Aufgaben zu (von 3 bis 6 Zug-Problemen). Um die Transformationsaufgaben in der vorgegebenen Anzahl von minimalen Zügen zu lösen, müssen Handlungsoptionen vorher im Kopf durchgegangen werden.

Der TL-D in dieser Version ist standardisiert und normiert. Es liegen Normierungen für Kinder und Jugendliche (Normstichprobe N = 299) im Alter von 6–15 Jahren vor sowie für Erwachsene (Normstichprobe N = 1263). Rohwerte sowie altersspezifische und bildungsspezifische Prozentrangwerte (PR) können somit ermittelt werden. Die Personen können Rohwerte von 0–20 erzielen. Dies entspricht der Anzahl der gelösten Aufgaben. Außerdem wird die Planungszeit protokollarisch erfasst. Für die Jugendlichen im Alter von 16 und 17 Jahren, für die keine gesonderten Normen vorliegen, wurde in dieser Untersuchung im Falle der 16-jährigen Jugendlichen die Normierung für 15-Jährige herangezogen und im Falle der 17-Jährigen sowie 18-Jährigen die bildungsspezifische Normierung der Erwachsenenstichprobe.

Objektivität:

Die Durchführungsobjektivität wird laut Testhandbuch (Tucha O. und Lange W. 2004) aufgrund der von ihnen vorgenommenen Standardisierung als gewährleistet beschrieben. Eine objektive Auswertung wird ebenfalls von den Autoren bestätigt.

Reliabilität:

Zusammenfassend ergeben sich gute bis zufriedenstellende Resultate bei der Überprüfung dieses Verfahrens auf Reliabilität (Tucha O. und Lange W. 2004):

a) Interne Konsistenz: Cronbachs Alpha = 0,785
b) Retest-Reliabilität: r = 0,861 (Halbtest-Reliablitätskoeffizient nach Spearman-Brown)

Validität:

- Inhaltsvalidität: In zahlreichen Studien wurde der „Turm von London" verwendet und dessen Sensitivität nachgewiesen. Eine Auflistung dieser klinischen Studien findet sich im Testhandbuch (Tucha O. und Lange W. 2004).

- Konstruktvalidiät: Der Zusammenhang zwischen dem Gesamtscore des TL-D und anderen kognitiven Leistungen wie allgemeine Intelligenz (Korrelation = 0,306), verbale Merkspanne (Korrelation = 0,297), verbales Arbeitsgedächtnis (Korrelation = 0,483), kognitive Verarbeitungsgeschwindigkeit (Korrelation = −0,509) und kognitive Flexibilität (Korrelation = −0,535) wurden anhand einer Teilstichprobe der Normstichprobe (n = 248) berechnet. Alle Korrelationen werden im Testhandbuch als statistisch bedeutsam (p < 0,01) berichtet. Es zeigte sich ein engerer Zusammenhang zur kognitiven Flexibilität (Korrelation = −0,535) und kognitiven Verarbeitungsgeschwindigkeit, die als exekutive Leistungen gesehen werden können. Auf der anderen Seite wird das im TL-D erfasste Merkmal nicht von anderen Verfahren erfasst.

Wisconsin Card Sorting Test (WCST; Heaton, Chelune, Talley, Chen, Kay & Curtiss 1993)

Der WCST wurde ursprünglich entwickelt, um die Fähigkeit zu abstraktem Denken und zur Änderung kognitiver Strategien in Reaktion auf veränderte Umweltkontingenzen zu erfassen (Berg 1948; Grant und Berg 1948, zitiert nach Heaton et al. 1993). Nach Luria (1973, zitiert nach Heaton et al. 1993) und Shallice (1982, zitiert nach Heaton et al. 1993) kann der WCST als Messinstrument der exekutiven Funktionen betrachtet werden, da die Fähigkeit zur Entwicklung und Beibehaltung einer angemessenen Problemlösungsstrategie und über verschiedene Reizbedingungen hinweg gefordert wird, um ein zukünftiges Ziel zu erreichen (zitiert nach Heaton et al.1993).

Der Untersucher legt bei diesem Testverfahren 4 Hauptkarten vor den Probanden, die sich in Form, Farbe und Anzahl der Symbole unterscheiden. Der Proband erhält dann nacheinander zwei Kartenstapel mit jeweils 64 Karten und muss jede Karte den 4 vorliegenden Hauptkarten zuordnen. Allerdings erhält der Proband keine Information, nach welcher Kategorie er dies tun soll. Nach der Zuordnung jeder Karte erfolgt vom Untersucher eine Rückmeldung, ob die Karte richtig oder falsch zugeordnet war. Dies soll dem Probanden helfen, die jeweilige Kategorie zu erkennen. Nach 10 durchgehend richtig gelegten Karten wird vom Untersucher ein Kategorienwechsel vorgenommen. Die neue Kategorie ist nun wiederum vom Probanden zu erkennen. Die Kurzversion besteht aus der Sortierung des ersten Kartenstapels mit 64 Karten. Dieser Test dauert laut Testhandbuch 20–30 Minuten.

Der WCST kann bei Kindern von 6 Jahren bis ins hohe Erwachsenenalter eingesetzt werden. Die Normierung erfolgte altersspezifisch von 6,5 Jahre bis 89 Jahre. Die Normierungsstichprobe bestand aus 899 Personen, wovon 453 Kinder und Jugendliche waren. Die Auswertung erfolgt nicht hinsichtlich einer Gesamtleistung; es werden 16 verschiedene Variablen erfasst, wie Anzahl der erkannten Kategorien, die gesamte Anzahl richtiger und falscher Antworten, ineffizientes Lernen, Perseverationen, Perseverationsfehler, Aufrechterhalten einer adäquaten Strategie, ineffiziente Konzeptualisierung.

Objektivität:

Die vorliegende Version ist bzgl. der Durchführung des Verfahrens und der Auswertung standardisiert. Zur Übereinstimmung der Auswertung zwischen verschiedenen Anwendern liegen einige Studien vor (Axelrod et al. 1992; Huettner et al. 1989, zitiert nach Heaton et al. 1993). Die Inter- und Intrascorer-Übereinstimmung wurden als exzellent beschrieben.

Reliabilität:

Die Autoren berichten eine moderate bis gute Reliabilität bei Kindern und Jugendlichen. Der generalizability coeffizient lag zwischen 0,39 und 0,72, mit einem Mittelwert von 0,57 und Median von 0,60.

Validität:

Der WCST wurde in zahlreichen Studien und bei sehr unterschiedlichen Gruppen eingesetzt. Viele der Studien werden im Testhandbuch aufgelistet und näher beschrieben. Insgesamt betrachten die Autoren die Validität des WCST zur Erfassung der Exekutivfunktionen bei neurologischen Patienten als nachgewiesen.

Behavioral Assessment of the Dysexecutive Syndrome (BADS; Wilson, Alderman, Burgess, Emslie, Evans, 1996)

Das Behavioral Assessment of the Dysexecutive Syndrome (BADS) beinhaltet sechs Untertests, mittels derer verschiedene Aspekte exekutiver Funktionen erfasst werden können. Es liegt eine deutsche Übersetzung vor (Ufer 2000). Die Beurteilung der Testergebnisse erfolgt anhand der englischen Normierungsstudie. Deutsche Normen liegen bislang nicht vor. Andere Länder haben bisher ebenfalls auf die englischen Normierungsdaten zurückgegriffen (Ufer 2000). Die englische Normierungsstudie bestand aus 216 Kontrollpersonen im Alter von 16 bis 87 Jahren (M = 46,6; SD = 19,8), der NART-IQ lag durchschnittlich bei 102,7 (SD = 16,2, Bereich 69–129).

Objektivität:

Aufgrund der Standardisierung der Testdurchführung und Auswertung sollte die Objektivität des Tests gewährleistet sein.

Reliabilität:

- Inter-Rater-Reliabilität: Die Inter-Rater-Reliabilität wird für alle 6 Untertests als ausreichend hoch angegeben (zwischen 0,88 und 1,00). Für 8 der 18 Parameter wurde eine vollständige Übereinstimmung gefunden. Eine Auflistung der Werte für alle 18 Parameter findet sich im Testhandbuch.
- Test-Retest-Reliabilität: Die Autoren der Testbatterie fanden einen klaren Trend zur Verbesserung der Testwerte in einer zweiten Testung, auch wenn der Unterschied der Mittelwerte nicht signifikant war (t > 0,05). Dies konnte in einer neueren Studie bestätigt werden (Jelicic et al. 2001).

Validität:

Zur Untersuchung der Validität des BADS wurden 78 neurologische Patienten mit dem BADS und einer Reihe von anderen Verfahren (dem WAIS-R; Wechsler 1981, dem Cognitive Estimates Test; Shallice und Evans 1978 und der Kurzform des Wisconsin Card Sorting Tests; Nelson 1976) untersucht. Im Vergleich der Patientenstichprobe mit der Kontrollstichprobe ergaben sich durch paarweise t-Tests signifikante Unterschiede der Gesamtprofilwerte der Gruppen (p < 0,0001). Die Kontrollgruppe zeigte nicht nur im Gesamtprofilwert deutlich bessere Punktwerte, sondern sie waren auch in jedem einzelnen Untertest signifikant besser als die Patienten. Der geringste Unterschied zwischen den Gruppen ergab sich für die Schlüsselsuche, der größte für den Modifizierten Sechs-Elemente-Test. Weitere Studien unterstützten die Anwendbarkeit und Nützlichkeit des BADS bei Patienten mit Schizophrenie (Ihara et al. 2000; Krabbendam et al. 1999), bei chronisch alkoholkranken Patienten (Moriyama et al. 2000) und bei depressiven Patienten (Paelecke-Haberman et al. 2005).

Behavioural Assessment of the Dysexecutive Syndrome for Children (BADS-C)

Vom BADS-C existiert eine britische, keine deutsche, Version.
Die Normen (N = 259) sind von 2003.
Numerische Angaben zu Reliabilität und Validität werden nicht gemacht. Zur Untersuchung der Validität wurden jedoch Vergleiche mit zwei anderen internationalen Testverfahren – Strenghts and Difficulties Questionnaire (SDQ) und Dysexecutive Syndrome Questionnaire for Children (DEX-C) – angestellt: „BADS-C would therefore seem to be a valid test of executive functioning in everyday life." (Manual) „BADS-C is a scientifically valid and reliable battery of tests of executive functioning for children and adolescents…" (Pearson Assessment). Durch Erfahrungen in der klinisch-psychologischen Anwendung des BADS-C schätzen die Leitlinien-Autoren, dass das Verfahren trotz mangelnder Überprüfung der Gütekriterien eine hohe klinische Validität besitzt.

5 Rechenfertigkeiten

Deutscher Mathematiktest DEMAT – basierend auf Lehrplänen der deutschen Grundschule

DEMAT 1+

Normierung:

- Deutschland 2000
- Alter: Ende der 1. Klasse bis Anfang der 2. Klasse
- Geschlechter getrennt

Reliabilität:

- Retest r = 0,65
- Interne Konsistenz:
  - 1. Kl. α = 0,89
  - 2. Kl. α = 0,88

Validität:

- Kriteriumsbezogen: Basisfähigkeiten Zahlenraum r = 0,77
- Lehrerbeurteilung r = 0,66
- Schnelligkeit Kopfrechnen r = 0,57

DEMAT 2+

Normierung:

- Deutschland 2001/2002
- Alter: Ende der 2. Klasse bis Anfang der 3.Klasse
- Geschlechter getrennt

Reliabilität:

- Interne Konsistenz
  - 2. Kl. α = 0,93
  - 3. Kl. α = 0,91
- Testhalbierung
  - 2. Kl. r = 0,95
  - 3. Kl. r = 0,94

Validität:

- Kriteriumsbezogen:
  - Mathematik-Note r = 0,66
  - Rechenhefte r = 0,66
  - Schnelligkeit Kopfrechnen r = 0,53
- Prognostische Validität:
  - Mathematik-Note 3. Kl. 0,67
  - Mathematik-Note 4. Kl. 0,64

DEMAT 3+

Normierung:

- Deutschland 2003/2004
- Alter: Letzte 6 Wochen der 3. Klasse bis erste 6 Wochen der 4. Klasse
- Geschlechter getrennt.

Reliabilität:

- Interne Konsistenz
  - 3. Kl. α = 0,83
  - 4. Kl. α = 0,81
- Testhalbierung
  - 3. Kl. r = 0,86
  - 4. Kl. r = 0,83
- Paralleltest
  - 3. Kl. r = 0,87
  - 4. Kl. r = 0,76

Validität:

- Kriteriumsbezogen: Mathematik-Note
  - 3. Kl. r = −0,68
  - 4. Kl. r = −0,50
- Prognostische Validität: Mathematik-Note
  - Ende der 4. Kl. r = −0,68
  - weitere Beschulung p = 0,60

DEMAT 4+

Normwerte:

- Deutschland 2003/2004
- Alter: 3 Wochen vor und nach Halbjahreswechsel der 4. Klasse bis 6 Wochen vor Ende der 4. Klasse
- Geschlechter getrennt.

Reliabilität:

- Interne Konsistenz
  - Mitte 4. Kl. $\alpha = 0{,}84$
  - Ende 4. Kl. $\alpha = 0{,}85$
- Paralleltest $r = 0{,}82$

Validität:

- Mathematik-Note Ende 4. Kl. $r = -0{,}7$
- Weitere Beschulung $p = 0{,}67$
- Heidelberger Rechentest $r = 0{,}72$

Zareki-K

Normierung:

- Deutschland und Schweiz 2007
- Alter: 5;0–7;5 Jahre
- Geschlechter getrennt

Reliabilität: $\alpha = 0{,}73–0{,}94$

Sensitivität: 68,5 %
Spezifität: 95,5 %

Zareki-R

Normierung:

- Deutschland und Schweiz 2006
- Alter: Klassen 1–4 (79–162 Monate)
- Geschlechter getrennt

Reliabilität: $\alpha = 0{,}93–0{,}97$

Validität: Kriteriumsbezogen:

- Lehrerbeurteilung: $r = 0{,}69$
- Mathematik-Note: $r = 0{,}64$

6 Lern- oder Merkfähigkeit

Verbaler Lern- und Merkfähigkeitstest (VLMT)

Die Normen stammen aus dem Jahr 2001 (n = 515).

Reliabilität:

Zur internen Konsistenz werden keine Angaben gemacht. Zur Untersuchung der Retest-Reliabilität wurde bei einer nicht näher beschriebenen Gruppe von 149 Patienten eine zweite Messung nach 8 bis 12 Monaten mit einer der beiden Parallelformen durchgeführt. „Retest-Paralleltestkorrelationen" zwischen den beiden Messungen wurden berechnet und darauf aufbauend kritische Differenzen für Leistungsveränderungen.

Validität:

- Summarisch werden faktorenanalytische Studien mit den VLMT-Variablen angeführt, auf die sich die Herausarbeitung der „Hauptvariablen" des Tests stützt und die die geringe klinische Relevanz der Fehlervariablen unterstreichen. Faktorenanalysen im Kontext von Testbatterien würden nahe legen, dass der Test sowohl „Kurz- als auch Langzeitaspekte" des Verbalgedächtnisses abzubilden vermag. Weiterhin wurde die Vergleichbarkeit von VLMT und ähnlichen international verwendeten Verfahren überprüft und bestätigt. In einer kleinen Vergleichsstudie mit 21 gesunden Kontrollprobanden zeigte sich, dass die zentralen Parameter des VLMT mit bildhaften Gedächtnisleistungen korrelieren, aber dass lediglich der erste Lerndurchgang (Dg1) mit Verfahren zum Arbeitsgedächtnis bedeutsam korreliert, nicht aber die „Hauptparameter".
- Klinische Validität: Schwerpunkt bilden Studien zur funktionellen Neuroanatomie. Der VLMT erwies sich als sensitiv für linksseitige mesiotemporale Funktionsstörungen, insbesondere eine verzögerte Abrufleistung. Temporo-kortikale Läsionen wirken sich stärker auf das Lernen bzw. die Aufnahme ins Langzeitgedächtnis aus.

Battery for Assessment in Children – Merk- und Lernfähigkeitstest für 6- bis 16-Jährige (Basic MLT)

Die Datenerhebung zur Normierung fand zwischen Februar 2005 und Juli 2006 statt (n = 405).

Die Reliabilität der einzelnen Skalen liegt zwischen 0,78 und 0,86.

Hinsichtlich der Konstruktvalidität erfolgten Validierungsstudien auf der Subtest-/Skalenebene über die Interkorrelationen der Subtestwerte und den Testskalen einerseits sowie über einen Stichprobenvergleich zwischen der Normstichprobe und einer klinischen Population andererseits.

Hinsichtlich der klinischen Validität wurden die diskriminanten diagnostischen Eigenschaften über den Vergleich der Normstichprobe mit einer klinischen Inanspruchnahmepopulation ermittelt. Dabei wurde deutlich, dass sich klinische und Normstichprobe signifikant voneinander unterschieden.

7 Aufmerksamkeit

Test d2 Aufmerksamkeits-Belastungs-Test (d2)

Normierung:

- Deutschland 2002, 9. Aufl.; neu normiert und überarbeitet; Re-Normierung 2000 („Eichstichprobe", N = 3176); insgesamt basieren die neuen Normen auf d2-Testergebnissen von mehr als 6000 Personen; ca. 2152 von 9–18 Jahren)
- Alter: 9;0–60;0 Jahre

Reliabilität:

Interne Konsistenz: Cronbachs Alpha: α = 0,95–0,98;

- Split-Half, Spearman-Brown: r = 0,95–0,98
- Guttman Split Half: r_tt = 0,95–0,98
    - Bezieht sich auf neue Normierung, Re-test r = 0,59–0,94
    - Bezieht sich auf ältere Studien mit alten Normierungen, keine neuere Erhebung

Validität:

- Konstrukt: signifikante Ergebnisse zwischen Lehrereinschätzung der Antriebsdimension (Aktivität) und Kontrolldimension (Willenskraft) und d2-Ergebnissen.
- Eine Übersicht über ältere Studien zum Zusammenhang zwischen d2-Variablen und konstruktkonvergenten Tests findet sich im Testmanual (S. 35), r = -0,71–0,78.
- Drei neuere Studien zur Konstruktvalidität liegen aus dem US-amerikanischen Sprachraum vor (Brickenkamp & Zillmer 1998), davon sind die beiden Studien von Culbertson zu beachten: Hier wurden Schulkinder und ADHD-Kinder untersucht; es ergaben sich signifikante Zusammenhänge bei Schulkindern: zwischen dem Turm von London (TOL) und dem GZ-F-Wert des d2 (r = -0,34– -0,44); bei ADHD-Kindern ergaben sich signifikante Zusammenhänge zwischen TOL (r = -0,45– -0,51) und GZ-F-Wert, zwischen Computerized Progressive Maze Errors (CPMZ) und GZ-F (r = -0,37), zwischen Controlled Word Association Test (COWA) und GZ-F (r = -0,45); keine signifikante Korrelation bestand dagegen zum Wisconsin Card Sorting Test (WCST).

- Es liegt eine etwas neuere Untersuchung zum Zusammenhang zwischen dem IST-2000 und d2 vor (1999/2000): Fast alle vergleichbaren Korrelationskoeffizienten weisen auf geringe, aber statistisch signifikante Zusammenhänge hin (r < 0,30).
- Weiterhin findet sich eine Auflistung älterer Studien im Testhandbuch (S. 38).
- Zur empirischen Validität liegen Studien aus dem Bereich: Verkehrspsychologie, ABO-Psychologie, Sportpsychologie, Pädagogische Psychologie, Umweltpsychologie, Psychiatrie, Neurologie, Klinische und Medizinische Psychologie, Experimentelle Psychologie sowie Pharmakopsychologie vor.

Intelligence and Development Scales IDS – Untertest „Selektive Aufmerksamkeit"

Normierung:

- Schweiz, Deutschland, Österreich 2007/2008
- Alter: 5;0–10;11 Jahre

Reliabilität:

Interne Konsistenz α = 0,57–0,96
Re-test r = 0,34–0,88

Validität:

- Konstrukt: bilden Entwicklungsschritte ab, Interkorrelation, Faktorenanalyse
- Kriteriumsbezogen: mäßige Korrelation mit HAWIK und Schulleistungstests
- Differenzierungsfähigkeit: Hochbegabte, Lernbehinderung, Fremdsprachigkeit, hyperkinetische Störung, Asperger Syndrom, Aggressive Verhaltensauffälligkeiten

8 Soziale Fertigkeiten oder Verhalten

Elternfragebogen über das Verhalten von Kindern und Jugendlichen (CBCL)

Deutsche Bearbeitung der Child Behavior Checklist (CBCL), 2. Aufl. mit deutschen Normen (n = 2888 bzw. für die Problemskalen 2856)

Normierung:

- Deutschland 1998
- Alter: 4;0–18;0 Jahre

Reliabilität:

- Interne Konsistenz: klinische Stichprobe: α = 0,94 (Gesamtauffälligkeitswert) bzw. α = 0,43–0,93 (für die Skalen), Feldstichprobe: α = 0,92 (Gesamtauffälligkeitswert) bzw. α = 0,21–87 (für die Skalen)
- Re-test r_tt = 0,72–0,89, für die Gesamtstichprobe r_tt = 0,81 (Remschmidt und Walter 1990)

Validität:

- Konstrukt: Faktorenanalysen
- Externale Validität vergleichbar mit der englischen Version und Versionen anderer Länder
- Diskriminante: Gesamtproblemwert sehr gut geeignet als Screening-Instrument; Skala „Aufmerksamkeitsprobleme" diskriminiert am besten zwischen Kindern/Jugendlichen mit und ohne Störungen.

Sensitivität für den Gesamtproblemwert als Prädiktor (Cut-off: T-Wert ≥ 60): 83,6 %.
Spezifität für den Gesamtproblemwert als Prädiktor (Cut-off: T-Wert ≥ 60): 83,9 %.
Sensitivität für den Gesamtproblemwert als Prädiktor (klinischer Range; Cut-off: T-Wert > 63): 69,7 %.
Spezifität für den Gesamtproblemwert als Prädiktor (klinischer Range; Cut-off: T-Wert > 63): 92,2 %

Youth Self Report (YSR)

Die Normierung erfolgte 1998 anhand einer umfangreichen bundesweit repräsentativen Stichprobe von annähernd 1800 Kindern und Jugendlichen.

Das Verfahren ist wegen seiner standardisierten Instruktion und Normierung objektiv in Bezug auf Durchführung, Auswertung und Interpretation.

Reliabilität:

Die Reliabilität der Syndromskalen konnte in einer klinischen Stichprobe (N = 292) weitgehend bestätigt werden: Für die Gesamtauffälligkeit und die Skalen „Internalisierendes Verhalten" und „Externalisierendes Verhalten" werden gute interne Konsistenzen von α = 0,86 festgestellt. Die Reliabilitäten der Syndromskalen „Aggressives Verhalten", „Angst/Depressivität", „Körperliche Beschwerden", „Dissoziales Verhalten" und „Aufmerksamkeitsprobleme" erweisen sich mit α = 0,70 als ausreichend.

Validität:

Die (faktorielle) Validität der Skalen wurde mittels Hauptkomponentenanalysen mit anschließender Varimax-Rotation anhand der 84 Items überprüft, aus denen sich die Syndromskalen zusammensetzen. Die Skalenbildung konnte in einer klinischen Stichprobe weitgehend bestätigt werden. Eine Ausnahme bildet dabei die Skala „Sozialer Rückzug", die jedoch schon in der amerikanischen Original-Stichprobe nicht faktoriell abgesichert werden konnte. Darüber hinaus ließ sich die faktorielle Struktur anhand konfirmatorischer Analysen in der deutschen Feldstichprobe genauso wie in 22 anderen Kulturen bestätigen.

Verhaltensfragebogen bei Entwicklungsstörungen (VFE-E)

Deutschsprachige Bearbeitung der Developmental Behavior Checklist (DBC) von Einfeld und Tongue; die an der deutschen Stichprobe durchgeführten Analysen findet sich separat (Steinhausen und Winkler 2005); die deutsche Normierung wurde an 721 Kindern und Jugendlichen ermittelt aus 75 Institutionen.

Normierung:

- Deutschland 2007
- Alter: 4;0–18;0 Jahre

Reliabilität:

- Re-test: ICC = 0,83–0,89 (deutsche Normierung)
- Interrater (Eltern): ICC = 0,80 (DBC: australische Normierung)
- Interrater (Veränderungssensitivität: DBC und klinische Beurteilungswerte): r = 0,86 (DBC: australische Normierung)

Validität:

- Inhalt: Krankengeschichten, Interviews, erfahrene Kliniker
- Konstrukt: Faktorenanalyse: interne Konsistenz am niedrigsten bei „Angst", Zuverlässigkeit dieser Subskala unbefriedigend, ansonsten für VFE-E gegeben: α = 0,58–0,90
- Diskriminante (Interkorrelationen der Subskalen sowie der 3 Grade der GB für VFE-E): überwiegend unter r = 0,60 (hinreichende Unabhängigkeit der Skalen), r = 0,17–0,69
- Differenzierungsfähigkeit: fetales Alkoholsyndrom, Prader-Willi-Syndrom, fragiles X-Syndrom, tuberöse Sklerose sowie Differenzierung zwischen Autismus und geistiger Behinderung (Steinhausen et al. 2004).
- Klinische Validität des DBC: überprüft an Autismus, Depression, Psychose, Hyperaktivität, Angst

Sensitivität für den DBC-Gesamtwert: 83 %
Spezifität für den DBC-Gesamtwert: 85 %

Strenghts and Difficulties Questionnaire (SDQ-DEU)

Deutschsprachige Bearbeitung der Strenghts and Difficulties Questionnaire (SDQ) von Goodman (die deutsche Übersetzung erfolgte 1997). Es existiert eine Elternversion, Lehrerversion und Selbstversion.
Die deutsche Normierung (Elternversion) wurde an 930 Eltern ermittelt.
Anmerkung: frei verfügbarer Fragebogen unter www.sdqinfo.org, hier finden sich Übersetzungen und eine Auflistung und Zusammenfassung bisheriger Publikationen.

Normierung:

- Deutschland 2002 (Elternversion)
- Alter 6;0–16;0 Jahre

Reliabilität:

- Cronbachs Alpha: α = 0,58–0,76 (einzelne Skalen)
- Cronbachs Alpha: α = 0,82 (Gesamtproblemwert)
- Es liegt eine zufriedenstellende interne Konsistenz vor (Klasen et al. 2003).

Validität:

- Inhalt: orientiert an älteren Fragebögen (Rutter) bzw. Faktorenanalysen längerer Fragebögen und nosologischen Konzepten
- Konstrukt: Faktorenanalysen: Bestätigung der englischen Skalen
- Kriteriumsbezogen: r = 0,68–0,82 (Skalen des SDQ und CBCL; Klasen et al. 2000)
- Klinische Validität: überprüft an einer klinischen Stichprobe (Becker et al. 2004)

Diagnostik-System für psychische Störungen nach ICD-10 und DSM-IV für Kinder und Jugendliche – II (DISYPS-II)

- Fremdbeurteilungsbogen/Selbstbeurteilungsbogen für den Störungsbereich ADHS (FBB-ADHS/SBB-ADHS)
- Fremdbeurteilungsbogen/Selbstbeurteilungsbogen für den Störungsbereich Störungen des Sozialverhaltens (FBB-SSV/SBB-SSV)

Es liegen Normen (offenbar aus dem Jahr 2000, genaue Angaben ließen sich nicht finden) für Fremd- und Selbstbeurteilungsbögen zur Erfassung von ADHS und Störungen des Sozialverhaltens vor.

Reliabilität:

Die Reliabilität der einzelnen Fragebögen kann mit Werten von α = 0,74 bis α = 0,94 als zufriedenstellend bis sehr gut bezeichnet werden.

Validität:

Die Konstruktvalidität wurde anhand von Faktorenanalysen überprüft und kann ebenfalls als zufriedenstellend bezeichnet werden. Da die Verfahren die Diagnose-Kriterien von ICD-10 und DSM-IV umsetzen, sind sie auch als inhaltlich valide anzusehen. Korrelationen zwischen Fremdbeurteilungsbogen, Selbstbeurteilungsbogen und Diagnose-Checklisten für ADHS, Störungen des Sozialverhaltens, Angst und Depression an Feldstichproben und klinischen Stichproben weisen außerdem auf eine gute konvergente und divergente Validität der Verfahren hin.

Intelligence and Development Scales IDS –
Untertests „Emotionen erkennen", „Emotionen regulieren",
„Soziale Situationen verstehen",
„Sozial kompetent handeln"

Normierung:

- Schweiz, Deutschland, Österreich 2007/2008
- Alter: 5;0–10;11 Jahre

Reliabilität:

- Interne Konsistenz α = 0,57–0,96
- Re-test r = 0,34–0,88

Validität:

- Konstrukt: bilden Entwicklungsschritte ab, Interkorrelation, Faktorenanalyse
- Kriteriumsbezogen: mäßige Korrelation mit HAWIK und Schulleistungstests
- Differenzierungsfähigkeit: Hochbegabte, Lernbehinderung, Fremdsprachigkeit, hyperkinetische Störung, Asperger-Syndrom, Aggressive Verhaltensauffälligkeiten

Register

A

Aarskog-Syndrom 58
Aggressivität 59
Alcohol related birth defect (ARBD) 11
Alcohol related neurodevelopmental disorder (ARND) 11
Alkohol-Exposition, intrauterine 56
Alkoholbedingte Entwicklungsneurologische Störung 11
Alkoholbedingter Geburtsdefekt 11
Alkoholkonsum, mütterlicher
– Prävalenz 26
– Risikofaktoren 30, 63
Alkoholspektrumstörung, Fetale 11
Alkoholsyndrom, Partielles Fetales 11
Anämie 57
Angststörung 59
Anlaufstelle, spezialisierte 40
Antikonvulsivum 58
Anwenderzielgruppe der Leitlinie 12
ARBD 11
ARND 11
Auffälligkeit
– faciale (des Gewichts) 44
– Wachstum 42
– ZNS 49
Aufmerksamkeit 49, 216
– Diagnostik, neuropsychologische 197
Aufmerksamkeits- und Aktivitätsstörung, einfache 58

B

Belastungsstörung, posttraumatische 59
Berufsverband, teilnehmender 15
Bildgebung 54
Bindungsstörung des Kindesalters, reaktive 59
Blepharophimosis-Syndrom 58
Body Mass Index 42

C

Child Behaviour Checklist (CBCL) 51
Chromosomenstörung 57

Confounder 18
Cornelia-de-Lange-Syndrom 58
Cytomegalie 57

D

Delinquenz 59
Di-George-Syndrom 58
Diagnostik
– bildgebende 54
– Empfehlungen 39
– neuropsychologische 196
Differentialdiagnose 57
Droge 57
Dubowitz-Syndrom 58

E

Einfluss, toxischer 57
Empfehlungsgrad 22
Encephalopathie, statische 11
Entwicklung 201
– Diagnostik, neuropsychologische 196
Entwicklungsstörung
– des Sprechens und der Sprache 58
– kombinierte umschriebene 58
– motorischer Funktionen 58
– schulischer Fertigkeiten 58
Entwicklungsverzögerung
– kombinierte 49
– konstitutionelle 57
Epidemiologie 60
Epilepsie 49, 52
– anderer Genese 59
Epstein-Barr-Virus (EBV) 57
Erkrankung
– chronische 58–59
– maternale 59
– renale 58
Evidenzbewertung 16
Evidenzklassifikationssystem nach Oxford 76
Evidenztabellen 79
Exekutive Funktionen 49
Exekutivfunktionen 197
Experten, teilnehmende 15

F

Fachgesellschaft, teilnehmende 15
Fähigkeit, räumlich-konstruktive 49
Fähigkeiten, räumlich-konstruktive 196, 204
Fehlbildungen 57
Feingold-Syndrom 58
Feinmotorik 49, 203
- Diagnostik, neuropsychologische 196
Fertigkeiten, soziale 49, 198, 217
Fetal alcohol spectrum disorder (FASD) 11
Fetales Alkoholsyndrom
- Diagnose 38
- Prävalenz 26
- Risikofaktor 35, 67
Formulierung von Empfehlungen 21
Funktionen, exekutive 49, 206

G

Geburts- oder Körpergewicht 42
Geburts- oder Körperlänge 42
Geburtsdefekt, alkoholbedingter 11
Geburtsgewicht 42
Geburtslänge 42
Geleophysic dysplasia 58
Genetische Syndrome 59
Gruppenprozess, nominaler 21
Gültigkeitsdauer 25

H

Hallermann-Streiff-Syndrom 58
Herpes simplex 57
Hirnschädigung, hypoxisch-ischämische 59
Human ImmundeJizienz-Virus (HIV) 57
Hypotonie 57

I

Implementierung 23
Infektion 59
- intrauterine 57
Intelligenz 198
- Diagnostik, neuropsychologische 196
Intelligenzminderung 58
- globale 49
Interessenkonflikte 25

K

Kabuki-Syndrom 58
Kleinwuchs
- familiärer 57
- psychosozialer 58
Kohortenstudie
- explorative 19
- nicht-konsekutive 19
Kollagenose 57
Komorbidität 57
Konsensfindung, formale 21
Kopfumgang 53
Körpergewicht 42
Körperlänge 42
Kriterium, konsentiertes 39

L

Leistungsfähigkeit, kognitive 196, 198
Leitlinie
- Finanzierung 25
- internationale diagnostische 18
Leitliniengruppe, Zusammensetzung 13
Lernfähigkeit 49, 215
Lidspaltenlänge 46
Lip-Philtrum-Guide 45
Literaturrecherche 16
- methodikfokussierte 60
- methodiksystematische 71
Literaturrecherche, fokussierte, Ergebnis 26
Literaturrecherche, systematische
- Ablauf 36
- Ergebnis 38

M

Magnetresonanztomographie (MRT) 55
Malabsorption 58
Mangelernährung 58
- postnatale 59
Mangelversorgung, pränatale 59
Merkfähigkeit 49, 215
- Diagnostik, neuropsychologische 197
Messung Körpermaß 42
Methodik 13, 76
Mikrocephalie 53
- familiäre 59
3-M-Syndrom 58

N
Nierenerkrankung, chronische 57
Nikotin 57
Noonan-Syndrom 58

O
Outcome-Kriterien 17
Oxford-Evidenzklassifikations-System 19

P
Panikstörung 59
Partial fetal alcohol syndrome (pFAS) 11
Parvovirus B19 57
Pathologie, fetale 57
Patientenvertretung FASD Deutschland e. V. 41
Perzentilenkurve, Lidspaltenlänge 46
Peters-Plus-Syndrom 58
Phenylketonurie, maternale 58
Plazenta praevia 57
Plazentation, gestörte 57
Präeklampsie 57
Prävalenz
– Alkoholkonsum, mütterlicher 26
– Fetales Alkoholsyndrom 26
Psychosyndrom, hirnorganisches 11

R
räumlich-konstruktive Fähigkeiten 49
Räumlich-visuelle Wahrnehmung 49
Reaktive Bindungsstörung 59
Rechenfertigkeit 49, 212
– Diagnostik, neuropsychologische 197
Röteln 57
Rubinstein-Taybi-Syndrom 58

S
Schädigung, toxische 59
Schlafstörung 59
SHORT-Syndrom 58
Silver-Russell-Syndrom 57
Skelettdysplasie 57
Smith-Lemli-Opitz-Syndrom 58
Soziale Fertigkeiten 49
Sprache 49, 202
– Diagnostik, neuropsychologische 196
Stereotypie 58

Stoffwechselerkrankung 57
Stoffwechselstörung 59
Störung
– affektive 59
– alkoholbedingte entwicklungsneurologische 11
– depressive 59
– hormonelle 58
– metabolische 57
Störung des Sozialverhaltens
– hyperkinetische 58
– mit oppositionellem aufsässigem Verhalten 58
– und der Emotionen 58
Strahlenexposition 57
Stress 57
Suchterkrankung 59
Syndrom, genetisches 57, 59

T
Teilbereich, neuropsychologischer 50
Teilnehmer am Leitlinienprojekt 14
Testverfahren
– neuropsychologische Güteparameter 198
– psychologische 52
Toluol 58
Toxoplasmose 57
Turner-Syndrom 57

V
Verabschiedung 23
Verbreitung 23
Verhalten, soziales 49, 198, 217
Verhaltensabweichung, sexuelle 59
Versorgung, gestörte intrauterine 57
Vitium, zyanotisches 57

W
Wachstumsauffälligkeit 42
Wachstumsstörung
– postnatale 57
– pränatale 57
Wahrnehmung, räumlich-visuelle 49, 196, 204
Williams-Beuren-Syndrom 58

Z
ZNS-Auffälligkeit, strukturelle 53
ZNS-Auffälligkeiten, funktionelle 49